365 DAYS OF LOW CARB RECIPES

Emma Katie

Copyright © 2016 Emma Katie

All rights reserved.

This book is licensed for your personal enjoyment only. This book may not be re-sold or given away to other people. If you would like to share this book with another person, please purchase an additional copy for each recipient. If you're reading this book and did not purchase it, or it was not purchased for your enjoyment only, then please return to your favorite retailer and purchase your own copy. Thank you for respecting the hard work of this author.

No part of this book may be reproduced in any form or by any electronic or mechanical means, including information storage and retrieval systems, without written permission from the author, except for the use of brief quotations in a book review. If you would like to use material from the book (other than just simply for reviewing the book), prior permission must be obtained by contacting the author at emma.katie@outlook.com.

Check out more books by Emma Katie at:
www.amazon.com/author/emmakatie

ISBN-13: 978-1539581376

Contents

Introduction 1

Appetizers 3

- Avocado Shrimp Salad in a Glass 4
- Fresh Mango Salsa 4
- Cheesy Stuffed Mushrooms 4
- Garlic Baked Camembert 5
- Sausage and Asiago Cheese Stuffed Mushrooms 5
- Fish Patties 6
- Upside-Down Tomato Frittata 6
- Vegetable Egg Muffins 7
- Spiced Pumpkin Seeds 7
- Herbed Ham Balls 8
- Sausage Stuffed Jalapeños 8
- Three Cheese Stuffed Jalapeños 9
- Crab Parmesan Dip 9
- Persian Cucumber Yogurt Sauce 10
- Roasted Garlic Cauliflower 10
- Prosciutto Wrapped Asparagus 10
- No Crust Spinach Quiche 11
- Garlicky Roasted Brussels Sprouts 11
- Bacon Wrapped Chicken Livers 12
- Chicken Nuggets 12
- Thai Mini Meatballs 13
- Bacon Wrapped Mozzarella Sticks 13
- Cream Cheese Stuffed Celery 14
- Caramelized Onion and Bacon Dip 14
- Jalapeño Lime Chicken Wings 15
- Grilled Portobello Caprese 15
- Bacon Wrapped Shrimps 16
- Parmesan Sesame Chips 16
- Eggplant Chips 16
- Zucchini Fritters 17
- Quiche Muffins 17
- Pistachio Goat Cheese Balls 18
- Tomato Mozzarella Towers 18
- Ceviche 19
- Pan Fried Asparagus 19
- Kale Chips 19
- Asparagus and Goat Cheese Frittata 20
- Crispy Roasted Asparagus 20
- Cottage Cheese and Bell Pepper Dip 21
- Asparagus and Ham Egg Cups 21

Prosciutto Chicken Wings 22
Salsa Cruda 22
Lemon Sautéed Brussels Sprouts 22
Cheese Fondue with Celery Stick 23
Loaded Cauliflower 23
Smoked Gouda Cauliflower Casserole 24
Green Beans with Bacon 24
Baked Mozzarella Sticks 25
Sesame Orange Shrimps 25
Balsamic Jumbo Prawns 26
Cheese and Spinach Stuffed Portobellos 26
Lobster Dip 27
Cilantro Sour Cream Dip 27
Quick Guacamole 28
Paprika Deviled Eggs 28
Baba Ganoush 28
Tomatillo Salsa 29
Bacon Cheddar Jalapeños 29
Fresh Herb Dip 30
Cucumber Salsa 30
Cream Cheese Stuffed Tomatoes 31
Four Cheese Broiled Tomato Slices 31
Caprese Salad Kabobs 32
Green Olive Zucchini Spread 32
Mexican Tomato Salsa 32
Ranch Dip 33
Goat Cheese Spread 33
Five Spice Glazed Pecans 34
Blue Cheese Cucumber Slices 34

Soups 35

Yam Creamy Soup 36
Spanish Tomato Soup 36
Cream of Spinach Soup 37
Truffle Cauliflower Soup 37
Cold Cucumber Soup 38
Creamy Cauliflower Soup 38
Thai Chicken and Mushroom Soup 39
Miso Soup 39
Creamy Asparagus Soup 39
Vegetable Soup with Cheese Topping 40
Butternut Squash Soup 41
Classic Chicken Soup 41
Creamy Mushroom Soup 42
Chinese Chicken Soup 42
Creamy Tomato Soup 43
Creamy Butternut Squash Soup 43
Vietnamese Beef Soup 44

Roasted Tomato Soup..44
Classic Chicken Soup with Egg Noodles 45

Salads...47

Mediterranean Calamari Salad 48
Grilled Chicken Salad 48
Artichoke Salad 48
Tomato and Lettuce Salad 49
Anchovy Salad Sauce 49
Tamarind Asian Salad 50
Asian Pork Salad 50
Onion Salad 50
Gravlax Fennel Salad 51
Tomato Cheese Salad 51
Egg and Cauliflower Salad 52
Kale Miso Salad 52
Green Olive Kale Salad 53
Caesar Salad 53
Spicy Vegetable Salad 53
Cress Salad with Sweet Chili Dressing 54

Main Dishes...55

Rosemary Salmon and Braised Broccoli...56
Tangy Scrambled Eggs 56
Fish Pockets with Sautéed Mushrooms 56
Breakfast from the West..57
Grilled Chicken with Buffalo Ranch Sauce 57
Sausage and Pork Bake 58
Egg Zucchini Casserole 58
Bacon Wrapped Duck Breasts 59
Bacon Wrapped Meatloaf..59
Onion and Sour Cream Pork Chops 60
Cranberry Muscadine Pork Roast...60
Vegetable Medley 61
Cheesy Squash Casserole 61
Indian Style Tofu 62
Sicilian Chicken 62
White Fish with Tomato Salsa 63
Chicken Paprikash 63
Tofu au Vin 64
Indian Spiced Chicken Stew 64
Cheese Stuffed Chicken Breasts 65
Cheesy Turkey Meatballs 66
Turkey Meatballs in Tomato Sauce 66
Cranberry Roasted Chicken 67
Steak with Mushroom Sauce 67
Steak and Spinach Salad 68
Chicken Cordon Bleu 68

Pork Chops with Creamy Sauce 69
Ham Stuffed Pork Tenderloin 70
Mustard Glazed Salmon 70
Chicken in Green Chile Sauce 71
Pork Chops in Marsala Sauce 71
Asian Style Steak 72
Garlicky Roasted Chicken 72
Braised Paprika Chicken 73
Butter Chicken 73
Herbed Beef 74
Beef Stroganoff in the Slow Cooker 74
Beef Carrot Stew 75
Beef Curry Stew 75
Slow Cooker Beef Roast 76
Ketchup Meatballs 76
No Bean Chili 77
Grilled Steaks with Eggplants 77
Beef and Portobello Stir-Fry 78
Red Snapper with Lychee 78
Fish Chili with Lemongrass 78
Thai Fish Cakes 79
Lamb Korma 79
Almond Cream Sauce Chicken 80
Grilled Jumbo Prawns 81
Cheesy Baked Chicken 81
Honey Glazed Chicken Thighs 82
Beef Ragu 82
Sticky Roasted Chicken 83
Spicy Roasted Chicken 83
Succulent Roasted Chicken 83
Caribbean Roasted Chicken 84
Vegetable Frittata 84
Seafood Tomato Stew 85
Green Salsa Chicken 85
Green Turkey Chili 86
Korean Style Chicken 86
Queso Chicken 87
Chicken Kabobs 87
Almond Crusted Chicken 88
Coconut Poached Salmon 88
Coconut Crusted Fish 89
Almond Crusted Fish with Leeks 89
Macadamia Crusted Lamb 90
Artichoke Frittata 90
Asian Style Patties 91
Asian Chicken Thighs 91
Mediterranean Style Salmon Fillets 92
Balsamic Glazed Lamb Cutlets 92
BBQ Chicken Burgers 93

BBQ Fish	93
Greek Omelet	93
Seafood Curry	94
Tomato Basil Haddock	94
Parmesan Eggplants	95
Tomato and Zucchini Stew	95
Cream Cheese Chicken	96
Poached Tilapia with Mayonnaise Sauce	96
Herb Crusted Salmon	97
Puff Pastry Wrapped Salmon	97
Baby Spinach Omelet	98
Rotisserie Chicken	98
Quick Zucchini Lasagna	99
Stuffed Bell Peppers	99
Cajun Jumbo Prawns	100
Cauliflower Chicken Curry	100
Pesto Chicken	101
Asian Slow Roasted Pork	101
Zucchini Pasta Bolognese	101
Lemon Zucchini Pasta	102
Shakshouka – Eggs in Tomato Sauce	102
Lettuce Wrapped Scrambled Tofu	103
Roasted Turkey with Paprika Butter	103
Asparagus Beef Stir-Fry	104
BBQ Ribs	104
BBQ Pulled Pork	105
Garlic Cheddar Chicken	105
Paprika Parmesan Chicken	106
Baked Halibut Fillets with Zucchinis	106
Italian Style Fish Fillets	107
Bacon Wrapped Pork Medallions	107
Burgundy Roasted Pork	108
Garlicky Roasted Pork Loin	108
BBQ Cumin Roasted Ribs	109
Blue Cheese Pork Chops	109
Onion Salmon Patties	110
Lemon Pork Loin Cooked in Oil Bath	110
Lemon Pepper Pork Chops	111
Ginger Pork Stir-Fry	111
Bacon Wrapped Pork Loin	112
Sausage and Zucchini Stew	112
Sauerkraut Pork Chops	113
Ham Cooked in Beer	113
Bacon Wrapped Pesto Chicken	113
Grilled Salmon with Wasabi Sauce	114
Marinated Grilled Tuna	114
Three Meat Meatballs	115
Grilled Pork Chops with Asian Style Sauce	115
Allspice Spare Ribs	116

Pork Chops with Sautéed Fennel ... 116
Carne con Chilies ... 117
Cajun Catfish ... 117
Poached Salmon with Piccata Sauce ... 118
Spicy Fried Cod ... 118
Roasted Trout with Yogurt Sauce ... 119
BBQ Slow Cooker Brisket ... 119
Grilled Salmon with Lemon and Tarragon Sauce ... 120
Blue Cheese Stuffed Pork Chops ... 120
Pepperoncini Beef ... 121
Cheeseburger Meatloaf ... 121
Beef Steak with Garlic Wine Sauce ... 122
Coffee Roasted Beef ... 122
Szechuan Beef ... 122
Sloppy Joe Casserole ... 123
Spicy Marinated Beef Steaks ... 124
Tomato Cabbage Stew ... 124
Cheesy Ham Quiche ... 124
Sherry Braised Beef ... 125
Cheesy Pork and Cauliflower Casserole ... 125

Side Dishes ... 127

Cauliflower Rice ... 128
Festive Sautéed Onions ... 128
Creamy Spinach ... 129
Roasted Cauliflower with Tomato Sauce ... 129
Almond Butter Broccoli Bake ... 129
Balsamic Grilled Zucchini ... 130
Lemon Sautéed Zucchini ... 130
Crispy Cabbage ... 131
Lemony Green Beans ... 131
Garlicky Spinach ... 132
Lime Drizzled Spinach ... 132
Balsamic Spinach and Onion Sauté ... 133
Italian Style Spinach ... 133
Garlic Mashed Potatoes ... 134
Cheesy Broccoli Casserole ... 134
Parmesan Zucchini Sticks ... 135
Fried Zucchini Slices ... 135
Sautéed Broccoli Rabe ... 136
Buttered Mushrooms ... 136

Desserts ... 139

Peach Cobbler ... 140
Coconut Almond Bread ... 140
Chocolate Walnut Candy ... 141
Orange Chocolate Truffles ... 141
Meringues ... 141

Carrot Cake Loaf 142
Mocha Chocolate Mousse 142
Orange Jelly Cheesecake 143
Coffee Granita 144
Orange Jelly 144
Quick Banana Ice Cream 144
Cheesecake Dessert Cups 145
Cinnamon Muffins 145
Blueberry Cream Cheese Pancakes 146
Ricotta Cheesecake 146
Pecan Scones 147
Mocha Cake 147
Coconut Bread 148
Lemon Curd 148
Key Lime Pie 149
Limoncello Cheesecake 149
Basic Crepes 150
Berry Cream Cheese Tart 151
Flourless Peanut Butter Cookies 151
Cream Cheese Raspberry Mousse 152
Chocolate Dipped Apricots 152
Flourless Brownies 152
Blueberry Ice Pops 153
Vanilla Orange Popsicles 153
Salted Chocolate Pecans 154
Double Berry Ice Cream 154
Pretzel Truffles 155
Strawberry and Yogurt Cups 155
Raspberry Panna Cotta 155
Quick Microwave Chocolate Cake 156
Peanut Butter Mousse 156
Pink Grapefruit Sorbet 157
Fudgy Brownies 157
Fresh Blueberry Tart 158
Frozen Bananas Covered in Chocolate 158
Watermelon Yogurt ice Cream 159
Mini Lemon Cheesecakes 159
Microwave Chocolate Lava Cake 160
Citrus Pound Cake 160
Almond Coconut Cake 161
Peanut Butter Cake 161
Raspberry Almond Crumb Cake 162
Ginger Cookies 162
Vanilla Butter Cookies 163
Spiced Cookies 163
Apple Cheesecake 164
Pecan Cookies 164
No Bake Cheesecake 165
No Crust Pumpkin Pie 166

No Crust Mocha Cheesecake ... 166
Chocolate Silk Pie ... 166
Coconut Crisp Cookies ... 167
Italian Ricotta Cake ... 168
Hazelnut Coffee Cookies ... 168
Cocoa Flax Cookies ... 169
Cottage Cheese Pudding ... 169
Minty Panna Cotta ... 170
Mocha Baked Custard ... 170
Coconut Panna Cotta ... 171
Chocolate Pots de Creme ... 171

Beverages ... 173

Chocolate Milkshake with Protein Powder ... 174
Chocolate Milkshake ... 174
Strawberry Almond Smoothie ... 174
Orange Creamsicle Smoothie ... 175
Cream Raspberry Sparkler ... 175
Spinach and Parsley Smoothie ... 175
Grapefruit Spinach Smoothie ... 176
Almond Apple Smoothie ... 176
Cinnamon Apple Smoothie ... 176
Avocado Spinach Smoothie ... 177
Kiwi Smoothie ... 177
Berry Spinach Smoothie ... 178
Savory Shake ... 178
Coconut Vanilla Shake ... 178
Green Smoothie ... 179
Berry Yogurt Shake ... 179
Banana Mocha Shake ... 179
Chilled Mango Smoothie ... 180
Kiwi Yogurt Shake ... 180
Vanilla Hot Chocolate ... 181
Mexican Hot Chocolate ... 181
Sugar Free Hot Chocolate ... 181
Spiced Hot Cocoa ... 182
Peanut Butter Smoothie ... 182
Grapefruit Kale Juice ... 182
Cantaloupe Yogurt Smoothie ... 183
Pineapple Milkshake ... 183
Nectarine Smoothie ... 183
Tropical Smoothie ... 184
Plum Tangerine Juice ... 184
Low Carb Lemonade ... 185
Pink Lemonade ... 185
Raspberry Yogurt Smoothie ... 185

Conclusion ... 187

Introduction

People are getting more conscious by the day about the food they eat. The saying "you are what you eat" seems to be as true as ever! The time of fast-food and unhealthy ingredients and foods is over! A new trend is rising and it involves healthy foods and healthy ingredient combinations, all for a healthier body and mind! Proteins and vegetables are no longer seen as the enemy, but as an ally to lean, strong muscles and a slim and fit body.

Tired of getting zero results with common, instant diets?! It's time for a change and you've come to the right place! This book focuses on one of the most realistic diets ever invented – the low carb diet. No more useless weight loss tips, no more calorie counting, no more starving! With the low carb diet none of that is needed! Instead, the low carb diet limits the amount of carbohydrates ingested and invests more in foods high in proteins and fat. The main purpose of this diet is weight loss, but it can benefit your body in terms of general health as well.

Carbohydrates, also referred to as carbs, are a type of calorie-providing macronutrient found in many foods and beverages. The main types of carbs are those found in grains, which are slow and hard to digest. But carbs are also found in fruits, vegetables, nuts and milk. However, these types of carbs digest more easily than the ones found in grains and are preferred over the ones found in grains.

Carbohydrates are the main source of fuel for your body. The carbs are broke down into sugars and starches then they are absorbed into the bloodstream where they spike the sugar level and reach the cells. When the sugar levels in your blood reach a high level, your body releases insulin which allows the cells to absorb sugars more easily. This, of course, leads to weight gain and that's exactly the opposite of what you want. The idea of the low carb diet is that decreasing the carbs also decreases the insulin levels and this process forces your body to burn fat for energy rather than use sugars as fuel. This means that having no more sugars to feed on, your system will begin to break down those stubborn fat cells in order to provide you with the much needed energy for your daily activities. Only then you can reach your goal – weight loss and therefore a better self-confidence, a healthier body and an improved mood.

A low carb diet focuses mainly on proteins – meat, poultry, fish and eggs – along with non-starchy vegetables and fruits, as well as dairy products. This diet generally excludes grains, legumes, breads, certain desserts, pasta, some nuts and seeds.

This book is the proof that a low carb diet is fun and includes delicious foods made using recipes that are easy to understand and follow. Exploring this book will reveal 365 amazing recipes, including appetizers, soups, salads, main dishes, side dishes, desserts and beverages. They are all easy to make and don't require any special cooking skills, except some chopping, greasing, heating, boiling and baking. You will see for yourself that cooking following the low carb guidelines is not as hard as it sounds, but it is incredibly rewarding, delicious and healthy!

Moreover, the recipes found in this book focus on healthy ingredients that offer a wide range of nutrients, from vitamins to minerals and antioxidants. I strongly believe that these recipes will improve your lifestyle and add nutritional value to your meals. Wait no more, it's time to lose those pounds and improve your life!

Low Carb Diet Focus Foods:

- Fish: halibut, cod, trout, salmon, herring, sardines
- Meat: chicken, turkey, duck, goose, quail, pork, beef, bacon, lamb, veal, venison
- Seafood: prawns, clams, mussels, shrimp, oysters, squid, crab

- Eggs
- Cheese: cream cheese, feta, mozzarella, Cheddar, blue cheese, Parmesan, Asiago, goat cheese, Swiss
- Vegetables: lettuce, celery, bok choy, arugula, chives, cucumber, fennel, mushrooms, pepper, radicchio, radishes, endives, artichokes, avocados, cauliflower, Swiss chard, onion, zucchinis, spinach, tomatoes, kale, leeks (should all be consumed with measure)
- Herbs and spices of all sorts
- Fats and oils: butter, olive oil, coconut oil, mayonnaise, canola oil, walnut oil
- Sweeteners: Splenda, Stevia, erythritol

Appetizers

Avocado Shrimp Salad in a Glass

Time: 30 minutes
Servings: 4-6

Ingredients:

1 pound fresh shrimps, peeled and deveined
Salt and pepper to taste
2 tablespoons olive oil
1 ripe avocado
2 tablespoons lemon juice
1 shallot, finely chopped
1 tablespoon chopped parsley

Directions:

1. Season the shrimps with salt and pepper and brush them with olive oil.
2. Heat a grill pan over medium flame and place the shrimps on the grill.
3. Cook them on both sides until golden brown.
4. For the sauce, puree the avocado with lemon juice in a blender.
5. Stir in the shallot and parsley then season with salt and pepper.
6. Mix the cooked shrimps with the avocado sauce and spoon the dish into cocktail glasses.
7. Serve immediately.

Fresh Mango Salsa

Time: 25 minutes
Servings: 4-6

Ingredients:

1 ripe mango, peeled and diced
2 green onions, chopped
¼ cup chopped cilantro
2 red bell peppers, cored and diced
1 jalapeno pepper, seeded and chopped
Salt and pepper to taste

Directions:

1. Combine all the ingredients in a bowl.
2. Mix gently and serve the salsa fresh.

Cheesy Stuffed Mushrooms

Time: 45 minutes
Servings: 6

Ingredients:

2 tablespoons olive oil
1 garlic clove, chopped
1 shallot, chopped
1 pound ground pork
Salt and pepper to taste
6 Portobello mushrooms
1 cup shredded mozzarella

Directions:

1. Heat the olive oil in a skillet and stir in the garlic and shallot.
2. Sauté for 2 minutes then add the pork and cook for 10 minutes, stirring often.
3. Add salt and pepper to taste then spoon the mixture into each Portobello mushrooms.
4. Top with mozzarella and cook in the preheated oven at 350F for 25 minutes or until golden brown and crusty on top.
5. Serve the mushrooms warm.

Garlic Baked Camembert

Time: 45 minutes
Servings: 4-6

Ingredients:

4 garlic cloves, minced
1 teaspoon dried rosemary
½ cup almond meal
1 pinch ground black pepper
1 medium size Camembert wheel

Directions:

1. Mix the garlic, rosemary, almond meal and black pepper in a bowl.
2. Place the cheese wheel in a baking tray and top with the almond mixture.
3. Cook in the preheated oven at 350F for 30 minutes.
4. Serve the cheese warm with seed crackers or veggie sticks.

Sausage and Asiago Cheese Stuffed Mushrooms

Time: 50 minutes
Servings: 8

Ingredients:

2 tablespoons olive oil
4 chicken sausages

365 Days of Low Carb Recipes

Salt and pepper to taste
16 medium size mushrooms
1½ cups grated Asiago cheese

Directions:

1. Heat the oil in a skillet.
2. Remove the casings of the sausages and place them in the hot oil.
3. Cook for 10 minutes then adjust the taste with salt and pepper if needed.
4. Spoon the sausages into each mushroom and top with cheese.
5. Cook in the preheated oven at 350F for 20 minutes or until golden brown and crusty.
6. Serve the mushrooms warm.

Fish Patties

Time: 45 minutes
Servings: 4-6

Ingredients:

2 pounds boneless fish fillets
2 garlic cloves, minced
¼ cup chopped parsley
¼ cup ground almonds
1 shallot, finely chopped
¼ cup grated Parmesan
1 egg
Salt and pepper to taste
Oil for frying

Directions:

1. Place the fish in a food processor and pulse until ground.
2. Stir in the garlic, parsley, almonds, shallot, Parmesan and egg then adjust the taste with salt and pepper and give it a good mix.
3. Wet your hands and form small patties.
4. Heat a skillet over medium flame and add a few tablespoons of oil.
5. Place the patties in the hot oil and fry on both sides until golden brown.
6. Serve the patties warm.

Upside-Down Tomato Frittata

Time: 30 minutes
Servings: 4-6

Ingredients:

6 eggs, beaten
1 tablespoon chopped chives
½ teaspoon dried basil
Salt and pepper to taste
2 tablespoons olive oil
2 tomatoes, sliced

Directions:

1. Mix the eggs, chives, basil, salt and pepper in a bowl.
2. Heat the oil in a skillet and place the tomato slices in the hot oil.
3. Cook for 2 minutes then pour in the egg mixture.
4. Lower the heat then top the skillet with a lid.
5. Cook for 10 minutes on low flame until the frittata is set.
6. When done, turn it upside down on a plate and serve it fresh.

Vegetable Egg Muffins

Time: 35 minutes
Servings: 12

Ingredients:

10 eggs, beaten
½ cup almond flour
1 teaspoon dried oregano
6 asparagus spears, chopped
2 red bell peppers, cored and diced
2 tablespoons chopped parsley
¼ cup crumbled feta cheese
Salt and pepper to taste

Directions:

1. Combine all the ingredients in a bowl.
2. Grease a muffin pan with vegetable oil then pour the egg mixture into the muffin cups.
3. Cook in the preheated oven at 350F for 20 minutes.
4. Let the muffins cool in the pan before serving.

Spiced Pumpkin Seeds

Time: 30 minutes
Servings: 4-6

Ingredients:

2 cups pumpkin seeds
1 teaspoon salt
½ teaspoon smoked paprika
½ teaspoon cumin powder
¼ teaspoon cinnamon powder
3 tablespoons olive oil

Directions:

1. Combine all the ingredients in a bowl.
2. Spread the seeds on a baking tray lined with parchment paper and cook in the preheated oven at 400F for 15-20 minutes.
3. Stir during the baking process a few times.
4. Serve the pumpkin seeds chilled.

Herbed Ham Balls

Time: 30 minutes
Servings: 4-6

Ingredients:

6 slices ham, finely diced
1 cup cream cheese, softened
3 green onions, chopped
½ cup grated Parmesan
Chopped chives for coating

Directions:

1. Combine the ham, cream cheese, green onions and Parmesan in a bowl and mix well.
2. Form small balls and roll them through chopped chives.
3. Serve the cheese balls fresh.

Sausage Stuffed Jalapeños

Time: 45 minutes
Servings: 6

Ingredients:

6 chicken sausage links
¼ cup grated Parmesan
12 jalapeño peppers

Directions:

1. Remove the casings from the sausages and place the meat in a bowl.
2. Add the cheese and mix well.
3. Carefully cut the top of the jalapeño peppers and remove the core and seeds.
4. Stuff the peppers with the sausage mix and place them in a baking tray.
5. Cook in the preheated oven at 350F for 25 minutes.
6. Serve the jalapeños warm or chilled.

Three Cheese Stuffed Jalapeños

Time: 45 minutes
Servings: 6

Ingredients:

½ cup cream cheese
½ cup shredded mozzarella
½ cup grated Parmesan

1 tablespoon chopped parsley
1 pinch salt
12 jalapeño peppers

Directions:

1. Mix the cream cheese, mozzarella, Parmesan, parsley and salt in a bowl.
2. Cut the top of each jalapeño pepper and remove the core and seeds.
3. Stuff the jalapeños with the cheese mixture and place them on a baking tray.
4. Cook in the preheated oven at 400F for 15 minutes.
5. Serve the jalapeños warm or chilled.

Crab Parmesan Dip

Time: 20 minutes
Servings: 2-4

Ingredients:

1 can crab meat, drained
½ cup cream cheese
½ cup mayonnaise

1 garlic clove, minced
½ cup grated Parmesan
½ teaspoon dried oregano

Directions:

1. Combine all the ingredients in a small bowl and mix well.
2. Serve the dip with vegetable stick or seed crackers.

Persian Cucumber Yogurt Sauce

Time: 15 minutes
Servings: 2-4

Ingredients:

2 cucumbers, finely diced
1 shallot, finely chopped
1 garlic clove, minced
1 cup plain yogurt
1 tablespoon chopped dill
Salt and pepper to taste

Directions:

1. Combine all the ingredients in a bowl and mix gently.
2. Season the sauce with salt and pepper and serve the sauce fresh.

Roasted Garlic Cauliflower

Time: 50 minutes
Servings: 4-6

Ingredients:

1 head cauliflower, cut into florets
4 tablespoons olive oil
½ cup grated Parmesan
1 teaspoon onion powder
1 teaspoon smoked paprika
½ teaspoon salt

Directions:

1. Place the cauliflower in a baking tray.
2. Drizzle florets with olive oil then sprinkle with Parmesan, onion powder, paprika and salt and mix to evenly coat them.
3. Cook in the preheated at 350F for 30 minutes.
4. Serve the cauliflower warm.

Prosciutto Wrapped Asparagus

Time: 40 minutes
Servings: 4

Ingredients:

12 asparagus spears
12 prosciutto slices

Directions:

1. Wrap each asparagus spear in a prosciutto slice and place them on a baking tray lined with parchment paper.
2. Cook in the preheated oven at 350F for 25 minutes.
3. Serve the asparagus warm.

No Crust Spinach Quiche

Time: 1 hour
Servings: 6-8

Ingredients:

2 tablespoons olive oil
1 shallot, chopped
1 garlic clove, minced
4 cups shredded spinach
6 eggs, beaten
½ cup almond flour
1 teaspoon dried basil
½ teaspoon salt
¼ teaspoon chili flakes
1 cup grated Cheddar cheese
1 cup grated Muenster cheese

Directions:

1. Heat the oil in a skillet and stir in the shallot and garlic.
2. Sauté for 1 minute then add the spinach and cook for 10 minutes until softened.
3. Remove from heat and let the mixture cool down slightly.
4. Stir in the eggs, almond flour, basil, salt and chili flakes.
5. Pour the mixture in a round quiche pan greased with butter.
6. Top with cheese and cook in the preheated oven at 350F for 40 minutes until golden brown and crusty.
7. Serve the quiche warm or chilled.

Garlicky Roasted Brussels Sprouts

Time: 45 minutes
Servings: 4-6

Ingredients:

2 pounds fresh Brussels sprouts, halved
1 cup cherry tomatoes
4 garlic cloves, minced
4 tablespoons olive oil
3 tablespoons lemon juice
1 teaspoon salt
1 teaspoon ground black pepper
½ cup grated Parmesan

Directions:

1. Combine the sprouts with tomatoes in a baking tray.
2. Mix the garlic, olive oil, lemon juice, salt and black pepper in a small bowl.
3. Drizzle this mixture over the sprouts and sprinkle with Parmesan.
4. Cook in the preheated oven at 350F for 25-30 minutes or until slightly golden brown.
5. Serve the sprouts warm.

Bacon Wrapped Chicken Livers

Time: 45 minutes
Servings: 10

Ingredients:

10 chicken livers
Bacon slices as needed

Directions:

1. Wrap each chicken liver into one or two slices of bacon, securing it with toothpicks if needed.
2. Place the wrapped livers in a baking tray and cook in the preheated oven at 350F for 25 minutes or until golden brown.
3. Serve the chicken livers warm.

Chicken Nuggets

Time: 45 minutes
Servings: 6-8

Ingredients:

4 eggs, beaten
1 cup almond flour
1 teaspoon salt
½ teaspoon cumin powder
½ teaspoon ground black pepper
4 chicken breasts, cut into strips
2 cups vegetable oil for frying

Directions:

1. Mix the eggs, almond flour, salt, cumin powder and black pepper in a bowl.
2. Add the chicken strips and mix to evenly coat them.

3. Drop a few strips in the hot oil and fry them until golden brown.
4. Remove them on paper towels and repeat with the remaining chicken strips.
5. Serve the nuggets warm.

Thai Mini Meatballs

Time: 40 minutes
Servings: 8-10

Ingredients:

1½ pounds ground beef
2 tablespoons coconut aminos
2 tablespoons Thai red curry paste
1 egg
¼ cup almond flour
1 teaspoon dried Thai basil
Salt and pepper to taste

Directions:

1. Combine all the ingredients in a bowl and mix them well.
2. Form small meatballs and place them all on a baking tray.
3. Cook in the preheated oven at 350F for 20-25 minutes or until fragrant and golden brown.
4. Serve them warm or chilled.

Bacon Wrapped Mozzarella Sticks

Time: 30 minutes
Servings: 8

Ingredients:

8 mozzarella sticks
1 egg, beaten
½ cup almond flour
8 bacon slices

Directions:

1. Dip each mozzarella stick into egg then roll it through the almond flour.
2. Wrap each stick into a slice of bacon and place them on a baking tray lined with parchment paper.
3. Bake in the preheated oven at 400F for 10 minutes.
4. Serve the sticks warm.

Cream Cheese Stuffed Celery

Time: 30 minutes
Servings: 8-10

Ingredients:

1 cup cream cheese, softened
2 tablespoons butter, softened
¼ cup crumbled goat cheese
1 teaspoon dried dill
1 tablespoon chopped chives
1 pinch chili flakes
6 celery stalks, cut into large chunks
Dill leaves, optional

Directions:

1. Mix the cream cheese, butter, goat cheese, dill, chives and chili in a bowl.
2. Take each chunk of celery and carefully stuff it with the cream cheese mixture.
3. Place on a platter and decorate with dill leaves if you want.
4. Serve fresh.

Caramelized Onion and Bacon Dip

Time: 35 minutes
Servings: 4-6

Ingredients:

2 tablespoons olive oil
4 bacon slices
3 red onions, sliced
1 cup cream cheese
¼ cup grated Parmesan
½ teaspoon garlic powder
Salt and pepper to taste

Directions:

1. Heat the oil in a skillet.
2. Place the bacon in the hot oil and cook until crisp then remove it on a platter and let it cool down.
3. Stir the onions into the fat left in the skillet and sauté them for 15 minutes, stirring often, until softened and slightly caramelized.
4. Remove from heat and let the mixture cool down.
5. Combine the onion with cream cheese, Parmesan and garlic powder then crush the bacon and mix it in as well.
6. Mix well then adjust the taste with salt and pepper.
7. Serve the dip chilled and fresh.

Jalapeño Lime Chicken Wings

Time: 1 hour
Servings: 4-6

Ingredients:

2 pounds chicken wings
2 jalapeño peppers, seeded and chopped
2 tablespoons coconut oil
2 tablespoons coconut aminos
4 garlic cloves, minced
1 lime, juiced
½ cup chopped cilantro
Salt and pepper to taste

Directions:

1. Combine all the ingredients in a zip lock bag and mix them well.
2. Marinate the chicken wings overnight.
3. The next day, place the chicken wings in a baking tray and cook in the preheated oven at 350F for 30-40 minutes or until golden brown.
4. Serve the chicken wings warm.

Grilled Portobello Caprese

Time: 40 minutes
Servings: 4

Ingredients:

3 ripe tomatoes, diced
1 garlic clove, chopped
4 basil leaves, chopped
1 tablespoon balsamic vinegar
Salt and pepper to taste
4 Portobello mushrooms
1½ cups shredded mozzarella

Directions:

1. Mix the tomatoes, garlic, basil and balsamic vinegar in a bowl. Add salt and pepper to taste then spoon the mixture into the 4 Portobello mushroom caps.
2. Top with shredded mozzarella.
3. Heat a grill pan or electric grill on medium.
4. Place the mushrooms on the grill and cook for 15-20 minutes until the cheese looks melted.
5. Serve the mushrooms warm.

Bacon Wrapped Shrimps

Time: 30 minutes
Servings: 6

Ingredients:

24 fresh shrimps, peeled and deveined
24 bacon slices

Directions:

1. Wrap each shrimp into one slice of bacon and place them all on a baking tray.
2. Cook in the preheated oven at 350F for 10-15 minutes.
3. Serve them warm or chilled.

Parmesan Sesame Chips

Time: 30 minutes
Servings: 4-6

Ingredients:

2 cups grated Parmesan
2 tablespoons sesame seeds

Directions:

1. Mix the Parmesan with sesame seeds in a bowl.
2. Drop spoonfuls of mixture on a baking sheet lined with parchment paper.
3. Bake in batches in the preheated oven at 400F for 5-7 minutes or until melted and slightly golden brown.
4. Let them cool in the pan before transferring on a platter.

Eggplant Chips

Time: 35 minutes
Servings: 2-4

Ingredients:

1 large eggplant
Salt and pepper to taste
¼ cup almond flour
1 teaspoon Italian seasoning
¼ cup grated Parmesan
2 tablespoons olive oil

Emma Katie

Directions:

1. Cut the eggplant into thin strips.
2. Season the eggplant slices with salt and pepper and place them in a baking tray lined with parchment paper.
3. Mix the almond flour with Italian seasoning and Parmesan then drop spoonfuls of mixture over each slice of eggplant. Drizzle with oil.
4. Cook in the preheated oven at 400F for 10-15 minutes and let them cool in the pan before serving.

Zucchini Fritters

Time: 30 minutes
Servings: 4-6

Ingredients:

2 young zucchinis, grated
¼ cup chopped parsley
1 egg
½ teaspoon cumin powder
¼ cup grated Parmesan
Salt and pepper to taste
¼ cup vegetable oil for frying

Directions:

1. Gently squeeze out part of the liquid found in the grated zucchinis and place them in a bowl.
2. Stir in the parsley, egg, cumin powder and Parmesan then add salt and pepper to taste.
3. Heat the oil in a skillet then drop spoonfuls of zucchini batter into the hot oil.
4. Cook on one side until golden brown then flip them over and fry on the other side as well.
5. Remove the fritters on paper towels and serve them warm.

Quiche Muffins

Time: 40 minutes
Servings: 12

Ingredients:

8 eggs, beaten
1 cup almond flour
½ teaspoon baking powder
2 green onions, chopped
6 asparagus spears, chopped
2 red bell peppers, cored and diced
1 carrot, grated
1 cup grated Cheddar

Salt and pepper to taste

Directions:

1. Combine all the ingredients in a bowl.
2. Mix well then adjust the taste with salt and pepper.
3. Pour the mixture into 12 muffin cups greased with oil or butter.
4. Cook in the preheated oven at 350F for 15-20 minutes.
5. Let the muffins cool in the pan before removing and serving.

Pistachio Goat Cheese Balls

Time: 30 minutes
Servings: 6-8

Ingredients:

6 oz. goat cheese
¼ cup cream cheese
1 tablespoon chopped chives
2 dried figs, chopped
½ cup finely chopped pistachio

Directions:

1. Mix the goat cheese with cream cheese, chives and figs in a bowl.
2. Form small balls and roll each of them through chopped pistachio.
3. Place on a serving platter.

Tomato Mozzarella Towers

Time: 15 minutes
Servings: 4

Ingredients:

4 basil leaves, chopped
3 tablespoons olive oil
2 tablespoons balsamic vinegar
8 slices mozzarella
8 slices tomatoes

Directions:

1. Mix the basil with olive oil and balsamic vinegar.
2. Layer the mozzarella with tomato slices on a platter.
3. Drizzle with the balsamic dressing and serve the dish fresh.

Ceviche

Time: 8½ hours
Servings: 4-6

Ingredients:

1½ pounds seafood (scallops, red snapper, halibut, prawns)
8 limes, juiced
2 celery stalks, sliced
4 tomatoes, chopped
1 sweet onion, finely chopped
Salt and pepper to taste
¼ cup chopped parsley

Directions:

1. Wash the seafood well and chop it. Place it in a bowl.
2. Add the lime juice and let the seafood soak up in the lime juice overnight.
3. The next day, drain well and stir in the remaining ingredients.
4. Add salt and pepper if needed and serve the ceviche fresh. Garnish with parsley.

Pan Fried Asparagus

Time: 35 minutes
Servings: 2-4

Ingredients:

¼ cup olive oil
2 garlic cloves, crushed
1 pound asparagus, trimmed
Salt and pepper to taste

Directions:

1. Heat the oil in a skillet and add the garlic. Cook until golden brown then remove the garlic and discard it.
2. Place the asparagus into the hot oil and cook, stirring often, for about 10 minutes.
3. Remove the asparagus on paper towels and sprinkle with salt and pepper to taste.
4. Serve the asparagus warm.

Kale Chips

Time: 35 minutes
Servings: 4-6

Ingredients:

8 cups shredded kale
4 tablespoons olive oil
Salt and pepper to taste
½ teaspoon smoked paprika

Directions:

1. Spread the kale in a baking tray.
2. Drizzle with olive oil and sprinkle with salt, pepper and paprika.
3. Cook in the preheated oven at 350F for 25 minutes and serve the chips warm or chilled.

Asparagus and Goat Cheese Frittata

Time: 30 minutes
Servings: 2-4

Ingredients:

4 eggs, beaten
4 asparagus spears, trimmed and sliced
1 shallot, sliced
Salt and pepper to taste
2 tablespoons olive oil
½ cup grated Swiss cheese

Directions:

1. Mix the eggs with asparagus and shallot. Add salt and pepper to taste.
2. Heat the oil in a skillet and stir in the egg mixture.
3. Cook on one side for 5 minutes then flip it over and cook for 5 additional minutes.
4. Top with cheese while still warm and serve immediately.

Crispy Roasted Asparagus

Time: 35 minutes
Servings: 4-6

Ingredients:

¼ cup olive oil
2 tablespoons lemon juice
1 pound asparagus, trimmed
1 cup almond meal
1 teaspoon dried Italian herbs
½ cup grated Parmesan

Directions:

1. Mix the olive oil with lemon juice in a bowl.
2. Add the asparagus and toss it around to evenly coat it.
3. Combine the almond meal with herbs and Parmesan.
4. Spread the asparagus on a baking tray and top with almond mixture, making sure each asparagus spear is well coated.
5. Cook in the preheated oven at 375F for 20 minutes.
6. Serve the asparagus warm and crispy.

Cottage Cheese and Bell Pepper Dip

Time: 20 minutes
Servings: 2-4

Ingredients:

4 roasted red bell peppers
1 cup cream cheese
1 red pepper, seeded
¼ cup grated Parmesan
1 tablespoon lemon juice

Directions:

1. Combine all the ingredients in a blender and pulse until smooth.
2. Spoon the dip in a bowl and serve it with vegetable sticks or seed crackers.

Asparagus and Ham Egg Cups

Time: 40 minutes
Servings: 12

Ingredients:

10 eggs, beaten
10 asparagus spears, trimmed and chopped
1 cup diced ham
1 teaspoon dried oregano
2 tablespoons chopped cilantro
Salt and pepper to taste

Directions:

1. Mix all the ingredients in a bowl.
2. Grease a muffin pan with oil then pour the mixture into each muffin cup.
3. Cook in the preheated oven at 350F for 20 minutes.

4. Let them cool in the pan before serving.

Prosciutto Chicken Wings

Time: 1 hour
Servings: 6

Ingredients:

12 chicken wings
12 slices prosciutto
Salt and pepper to taste

Directions:

1. Cut and trim the chicken wings then wrap each wing in one slice of prosciutto.
2. Place the wings in a baking tray lined with parchment paper and cook in the preheated oven at 350F for 20-30 minutes.
3. Let them cool slightly before serving.

Salsa Cruda

Time: 25 minutes
Servings: 2-4

Ingredients:

2 ripe tomatoes, diced
1 cucumber, diced
½ celery stalk, diced
1 garlic clove, minced
¼ cup chopped cilantro

¼ cup chopped parsley
1 lime, juiced
1 red pepper, chopped
Salt and pepper to taste

Directions:

1. Combine all the ingredients in a bowl and mix gently.
2. Season with salt and pepper and serve the salsa fresh.

Lemon Sautéed Brussels Sprouts

Time: 45 minutes
Servings: 4-6

Ingredients:

4 tablespoons olive oil
1 shallot, chopped
2 pounds Brussels sprouts, halved
1 lemon, juiced
Salt and pepper to taste

Directions:

1. Heat the oil in a skillet and stir in the shallot.
2. Sauté for 2 minutes then add the sprouts.
3. Drizzle with lemon juice and lower the heat. Cook for 20 minutes, stirring often.
4. Add salt and pepper to taste. Serve the sprouts warm.

Cheese Fondue with Celery Stick

Time: 35 minutes
Servings: 6-8

Ingredients:

1 cup heavy cream
1 cup grated Cheddar
1 cup shredded mozzarella
1 cup smoked Gouda
4 celery stalks, cut into sticks

Directions:

1. Bring the heavy cream to the boiling point in a heavy saucepan.
2. Remove from heat and stir in the three cheeses.
3. Mix until smooth and creamy.
4. Serve the fondue warm by dipping celery stick into the melted cheese mix.

Loaded Cauliflower

Time: 1 hour
Servings: 4-6

Ingredients:

2 tablespoons butter
4 bacon slices, chopped
1 cup cream cheese
1 head cauliflower, cut into florets
½ cup breadcrumbs
1½ cups grated mozzarella
½ cup grated Cheddar

Directions:

1. Melt the butter in a skillet and stir in the bacon.
2. Cook until crisp then remove from heat and stir in the cream cheese.
3. Add the cauliflower florets and mix until evenly coated.
4. Transfer the cauliflower in a deep dish baking pan and top with breadcrumbs followed by cheese.
5. Cook in the preheated oven at 350F for 35-40 minutes or until crusty and golden brown.
6. Serve the dish warm.

Smoked Gouda Cauliflower Casserole

Time: 1 hour
Servings: 4-6

Ingredients:

4 bacon slices, chopped
1 sweet onion, sliced
1 garlic clove, minced
½ cup cream cheese
1 head cauliflower, cut into florets
1½ cups grated smoked Gouda cheese

Directions:

1. Heat a skillet over medium flame.
2. Stir in the bacon and cook until crisp.
3. Stir in the onion and garlic and sauté for 2 minutes.
4. Remove from heat and stir in the cream cheese. Mix until melted.
5. Add the cauliflower and mix to evenly coat it then transfer it in a deep dish baking pan.
6. Top with cheese and cook in the preheated oven at 350F for 30-40 minutes.
7. Serve the casserole warm.

Green Beans with Bacon

Time: 35 minutes
Servings: 2-4

Ingredients:

1½ pounds green beans
2 tablespoons olive oil
6 bacon slices, cut into thin strips
¼ cup grated Parmesan

Directions:

1. Pour a few cups of water in a large pot and bring it to a boil.
2. Throw in the green beans and cook them for 10 minutes.
3. Heat the oil in a skillet and stir in the bacon strips.
4. Cook until crisp then add the drained beans.
5. Cook 10 additional minutes, stirring often, then remove from heat and sprinkle with Parmesan before serving.

Baked Mozzarella Sticks

Time: 45 minutes
Servings: 6

Ingredients:

½ cup almond meal
½ cup breadcrumbs
1 teaspoon dried Italian herbs

12 mozzarella sticks
2 eggs, beaten

Directions:

1. Mix the almond meal with breadcrumbs and herbs in a bowl.
2. Dip the mozzarella sticks into egg then roll them through breadcrumbs and place them on a baking tray lined with parchment paper.
3. Cook in the preheated oven at 400F for 15-20 minutes.
4. Serve the mozzarella sticks warm.

Sesame Orange Shrimps

Time: 45 minutes
Servings: 4-6

Ingredients:

¼ cup soy sauce
1 teaspoon sesame oil
1 tablespoon cornstarch
¼ teaspoon red pepper flakes
2 tablespoons orange juice
2 tablespoons sesame seeds
1½ pounds fresh shrimp, peeled and deveined

2 green onions, chopped

Directions:

1. Mix the soy sauce, sesame oil, cornstarch, red pepper flakes, orange juice and sesame seeds in a bowl.
2. Place the shrimps on wooden skewers then dip them in the mixture you made earlier.
3. Heat a grill pan over medium flame and place the skewers on the grill.
4. Cook on both sides until golden brown.
5. Serve the shrimps warm, topped with green onions.

Balsamic Jumbo Prawns

Time: 30 minutes
Servings: 4-6

Ingredients:

½ cup balsamic vinegar
1 teaspoon salt
1 teaspoon chili flakes

1½ pounds jumbo prawns
Wooden skewers

Directions:

1. Mix the balsamic vinegar with salt and chili flakes in a bowl.
2. Add the prawns and let them marinate for 10 minutes.
3. Place the prawns on wooden skewers.
4. Heat a grill pan over medium to high flame and place the prawns on the grill.
5. Cook them on both sides until golden brown and serve the prawns warm.

Cheese and Spinach Stuffed Portobellos

Time: 1 hour
Servings: 6

Ingredients:

2 tablespoons olive oil
1 garlic clove, minced
1 shallot, chopped
10 oz. spinach, shredded
Salt and pepper to taste
6 Portobello mushrooms
1 cup shredded mozzarella

½ cup grated Parmesan

Directions:

1. Heat the oil in a skillet and stir in the garlic and shallot.
2. Cook for 2-3 minutes until soft then stir in the spinach and sauté for 5 minutes. Add salt and pepper to taste.
3. Remove from heat and spoon the mixture into your Portobello mushrooms.
4. Top with Parmesan and mozzarella and place the mushrooms in a baking pan.
5. Cook in the preheated oven at 350F for 20-25 minutes.
6. Serve the mushrooms warm.

Lobster Dip

Time: 15 minutes
Servings: 2-4

Ingredients:

1 can lobster meat, drained
1 green onion, chopped
1 cup cream cheese, softened
2 tablespoons melted butter
1 teaspoon lemon juice
1 teaspoon prepared horseradish
Salt and pepper to taste

Directions:

1. Combine all the ingredients in a bowl and mix well.
2. Serve the dip fresh, with vegetable sticks or seed crackers.

Cilantro Sour Cream Dip

Time: 15 minutes
Servings: 2-4

Ingredients:

1 cup sour cream
½ cup cream cheese
½ cup finely chopped cilantro
¼ teaspoon cumin powder
1 tablespoon lemon juice
Salt and pepper to taste

Directions:

1. Combine all the ingredients in a bowl.
2. Mix well then season with salt and pepper to taste.
3. Serve the dip fresh.

Quick Guacamole

Time: 20 minutes
Servings: 2-4

Ingredients:

1 ripe avocado, mashed
1 lime, juiced
1 shallot, finely chopped
¼ cup chopped cilantro

2 ripe tomatoes, diced
1 garlic clove, minced
Salt and pepper to taste

Directions:

1. Combine all the ingredients in a bowl.
2. Mix well then season with salt and pepper.
3. Serve the guacamole as fresh as possible.

Paprika Deviled Eggs

Time: 40 minutes
Servings: 6

Ingredients:

6 eggs
¼ cup mayonnaise
1 teaspoon smoked paprika

1 tablespoon chopped chives
Salt and pepper to taste

Directions:

1. Boil the eggs for 10 minutes until hard then carefully peel them and slice them in half lengthwise.
2. Remove the egg yolks in a bowl and mash them well with a fork.
3. Stir in the mayonnaise, paprika and chives then season with salt and pepper.
4. Spoon the filling back into the egg white halves and place on a platter.
5. Serve the eggs fresh.

Baba Ganoush

Time: 40 minutes
Servings: 2-4

Ingredients:

1 eggplant
¼ cup tahini paste
2 garlic cloves, minced
½ shallot, finely chopped

Salt and pepper to taste
1 tablespoon lemon juice
2 tablespoons olive oil

Directions:

1. Cut the eggplant in half lengthwise and place the halves on a baking tray.
2. Cook in the preheated oven at 375F for 30 minutes until softened.
3. Scoop out the soft flesh and mash it well in a blender.
4. Stir in the remaining ingredients and mix well.
5. Serve the baba ganoush fresh.

Tomatillo Salsa

Time: 35 minutes
Servings: 4-6

Ingredients:

6 tomatillos, husked
1 shallot, chopped
2 garlic cloves, minced
2 jalapeno peppers, seeded and chopped

¼ cup finely chopped cilantro
1 tablespoon olive oil
Salt and pepper to taste

Directions:

1. Place the tomatillos in a saucepan and cover them with water.
2. Bring to a boil and cook for 10 minutes then drain and place them in a food processor.
3. Pulse the tomatillos until smooth then transfer the mixture into a bowl and stir in the next five ingredients.
4. Season with salt and pepper and serve the salsa as fresh as possible.

Bacon Cheddar Jalapeños

Time: 30 minutes
Servings: 12

Ingredients:

2 cups grated Cheddar cheese

365 Days of Low Carb Recipes

½ cup cream cheese
1 teaspoon dried oregano
6 large jalapeño peppers, halved and cored
12 slices bacon

Directions:

1. Mix the Cheddar with cream cheese and oregano in a bowl.
2. Spoon the cheese mixture into the jalapeño halves then wrap each pepper half into a bacon slice.
3. Place the jalapeño halves in a baking tray lined with parchment paper and cook in the preheated oven at 400F for 10 minutes.
4. Serve the jalapeños warm.

Fresh Herb Dip

Time: 15 minutes
Servings: 2-4

Ingredients:

½ cup mayonnaise
½ cup sour cream
2 tablespoons chopped parsley
2 tablespoons chopped cilantro
1 tablespoon chopped chives
1 tablespoon lemon juice
¼ teaspoon garlic powder
Salt and pepper to taste

Directions:

1. Combine all the ingredients in a bowl and mix well.
2. Adjust the taste with salt and pepper and serve the dip fresh.

Cucumber Salsa

Time: 20 minutes
Servings: 4-6

Ingredients:

2 large cucumbers, peeled and diced
1 ripe tomato, seeded and diced
1 shallot, finely chopped
2 tablespoons chopped parsley
1 jalapeño pepper, chopped
1 garlic clove, minced
1 lime, juiced
Salt and pepper to taste

Directions:

1. Combine all the ingredients in a bowl.
2. Add salt and pepper to taste and serve the salsa as fresh as possible.

Cream Cheese Stuffed Tomatoes

Time: 25 minutes
Servings: 6

Ingredients:

6 medium size tomatoes
1½ cups cream cheese
1 tablespoon chopped chives
2 tablespoons chopped parsley
1 pinch chili powder
Salt and pepper to taste

Directions:

1. Cut the top of each tomato and carefully remove the flesh, making sure to preserve the skins intact.
2. Mix the cream cheese, chives, parsley and chili powder in a bowl and add salt and pepper to taste.
3. Spoon the cream cheese mixture into the tomatoes and decorate with a leaf of parsley.
4. Serve the stuffed tomatoes fresh.

Four Cheese Broiled Tomato Slices

Time: 25 minutes
Servings: 4-6

Ingredients:

½ cup grated Parmesan
1 cup shredded mozzarella
½ cup grated Cheddar
½ cup ricotta cheese
1 teaspoon dried Italian herbs
¼ teaspoon garlic powder
Salt and pepper to taste
3 ripe tomatoes, cut into thick slices

Directions:

1. Mix the Parmesan, mozzarella, Cheddar and ricotta in a bowl.
2. Add the herbs, garlic powder, salt and pepper and mix well.
3. Place the tomato slices on a baking tray lined with parchment paper.

4. Top each slice with a dollop of cheese mixture and cook under the broiler for 5-7 minutes or until golden brown and crusty on top.
5. Serve the tomato slices warm or chilled.

Caprese Salad Kabobs

Time: 30 minutes
Servings: 6-8

Ingredients:

3 cups cherry tomatoes
2 cups cherry-size mozzarella balls, drained
½ cup fresh basil leaves
Salt and pepper to taste
2 tablespoons balsamic vinegar

Directions:

1. Layer the tomatoes, mozzarella and basil leaves on wooden skewers.
2. Sprinkle with salt and pepper and drizzle with balsamic vinegar just before serving.

Green Olive Zucchini Spread

Time: 20 minutes
Servings: 4-6

Ingredients:

1½ cups cream cheese
½ cup green olives, pitted
½ cup chopped parsley
2 garlic cloves
1 shallot, chopped
1 young zucchini, grated
Salt and pepper to taste

Directions:

1. Mix the cream cheese, green olives, parsley and garlic in a food processor and pulse until smooth.
2. Stir in the shallot, zucchini, salt and pepper and mix well.
3. Serve the spread fresh.

Mexican Tomato Salsa

Time: 20 minutes
Servings: 4-6

Ingredients:

- 4 ripe tomatoes, diced
- 1 red onion, finely chopped
- 4 jalapeño peppers, seeded and chopped
- 2 garlic cloves, minced
- ½ cup chopped cilantro
- Salt and pepper to taste

Directions:

1. Combine all the ingredients in a bowl.
2. Season with salt and pepper and serve the salsa fresh.

Ranch Dip

Time: 15 minutes
Servings: 2-4

Ingredients:

- ½ cup mayonnaise
- ½ cup ranch salad dressing
- ½ cup low fat sour cream
- ¼ cup grated Parmesan cheese
- 4 bacon slices, cooked and shredded
- ½ teaspoon dried basil

Directions:

1. Combine all the ingredients in a bowl and mix well.
2. Serve the dip with vegetable sticks.

Goat Cheese Spread

Time: 15 minutes
Servings: 4-6

Ingredients:

- 1 cup crumbled goat cheese
- ½ cup low fat mayonnaise
- 1 apple, diced
- 1 pinch ground black pepper
- Seed crackers for serving

Directions:

1. Combine all the ingredients in a bowl and mix well.
2. Spread the goat cheese mixture over seed crackers and serve fresh.

365 Days of Low Carb Recipes

Five Spice Glazed Pecans

Time: 30 minutes
Servings: 4-6

Ingredients:

2 cups pecan halves
3 tablespoons melted butter
2 tablespoons brown sugar
1½ teaspoons five spice powder
½ teaspoon salt

Directions:

1. Mix the pecans with butter in a bowl and toss them around to evenly coat them.
2. Sprinkle with sugar, powder and salt and mix well.
3. Spread the pecans on a baking tray lined with parchment paper and cook in the preheated oven at 350F for 15-20 minutes or until golden brown and crisp.
4. Let them cool in the pan before serving.

Blue Cheese Cucumber Slices

Time: 20 minutes
Servings: 6-8

Ingredients:

1 cup crumbled blue cheese
¼ cup cream cheese
2 cucumbers, cut into thick slices
¼ cup chopped walnuts

Directions:

1. Mix the blue cheese with cream cheese in a bowl.
2. Drop spoonfuls of blue cheese mixture over each slice of cucumber. Top with walnuts and serve them fresh.

Soups

Yam Creamy Soup

Time: 1 hour
Servings: 4-6

Ingredients:

2 tablespoons olive oil
1 shallot, chopped
1 garlic clove, minced
4 yams, peeled and cubed

1 cup chicken stock
3 cups water
½ teaspoon dried sage
Salt and pepper to taste

Directions:

1. Heat the oil in a soup pot and stir in the shallot and garlic.
2. Sauté for 2 minutes then add the yams, stock and water, as well as the dried sage.
3. Adjust the taste with salt and pepper and cook over medium flame for 25 minutes.
4. Puree the soup with an immersion blender and serve the soup warm.

Spanish Tomato Soup

Time: 30 minutes
Servings: 4-6

Ingredients:

6 ripe tomatoes, peeled and seeded
2 cucumbers, peeled
2 roasted bell peppers
1 garlic clove, peeled
1 shallot

1 cup water
½ teaspoon chili powder
Salt and pepper to taste
Chopped herbs for serving

Directions:

1. Combine the tomatoes, cucumbers, bell peppers, garlic, shallot and water in a blender and pulse until smooth.
2. Stir in the chili powder, salt and pepper and serve the soup fresh, topped with freshly chopped herbs.

Cream of Spinach Soup

Time: 1 hour
Servings: 4-6

Ingredients:

2 tablespoons butter
2 garlic cloves, chopped
1 sweet onion, chopped
½ celery stalk, sliced
4 cups shredded spinach
4 cups chicken stock
Salt and pepper to taste
½ cup sour cream
½ cup heavy cream

Directions:

1. Melt the butter in a soup pot and stir in the garlic and onion.
2. Sauté for 2 minutes then stir in the celery and spinach.
3. Add the stock and cook the soup for 20 minutes.
4. Puree the soup with an immersion blender then stir in the sour cream and heavy cream and mix well.
5. Season with salt and pepper and serve the soup warm.

Truffle Cauliflower Soup

Time: 40 minutes
Servings: 4-6

Ingredients:

2 tablespoons olive oil
2 leeks, sliced
1 head cauliflower, cut into florets
2 cups chicken stock
2 cups water
1 pinch nutmeg
1 cup heavy cream
1 teaspoon truffle oil
Salt and pepper to taste

Directions:

1. Heat the olive oil in a soup pot and stir in the leeks.
2. Sauté for 5 minutes until soft then add the cauliflower, stock, water and nutmeg.
3. Cook the soup for 20 minutes then puree the soup with an immersion blender until smooth.
4. Stir in the heavy cream and truffle oil, then adjust the taste with salt and pepper and serve the soup warm.

Cold Cucumber Soup

Time: 20 minutes
Servings: 2-4

Ingredients:

4 cucumbers, peeled and sliced
2 cups plain yogurt
1 cup buttermilk
2 tablespoons olive oil
Salt and pepper to taste
2 tablespoons chopped chives
1 teaspoon chopped dill
Ice cubes for serving

Directions:

1. Combine the cucumbers, yogurt, buttermilk and olive oil in a blender and pulse until smooth.
2. Add salt and pepper to taste. Stir in the chives and dill and pour the soup into serving bowls.
3. Top with ice cubes before serving.

Creamy Cauliflower Soup

Time: 40 minutes
Servings: 4-6

Ingredients:

2 tablespoons olive oil
2 garlic cloves, minced
1 shallot, chopped
1 head cauliflower, cut into florets
4 cups vegetable stock
2 cups water
Salt and pepper to taste
1 cup heavy cream
1 pinch nutmeg
½ cup grated Cheddar

Directions:

1. Heat the olive oil in a soup pot and stir in the garlic and shallot.
2. Sauté for 2 minutes then stir in the cauliflower, stock and water.
3. Season with salt and pepper to taste and cook over medium flame for 25 minutes.
4. Puree the soup with an immersion blender then stir in the cream and nutmeg.
5. Serve the soup warm, topped with cheese.

Thai Chicken and Mushroom Soup

Time: 40 minutes
Servings: 4-6

Ingredients:

6 cups chicken stock
2 cups shredded chicken
2 cups sliced mushrooms
2 tablespoons Thai red curry paste

1 teaspoon fish sauce
1 lime, juiced
3 green onions, sliced

Directions:

1. Combine the stock, chicken, mushrooms, curry paste and fish sauce in a soup pot.
2. Cook on low heat for 20 minutes then remove from heat and stir in the lime juice and green onions.
3. Serve the soup warm.

Miso Soup

Time: 35 minutes
Servings: 4-6

Ingredients:

6 cups water
2 tablespoons dashi granules
2 cups cubed tofu
2 tablespoons dried seaweed, chopped

2 tablespoons soy sauce
¼ cup miso paste
2 green onions, chopped

Directions:

1. Combine the water, dashi granules, tofu, seaweed and soy sauce in a soup pot.
2. Bring to a boil and cook for 10 minutes.
3. Stir in the miso paste and remove from heat.
4. Add the green onions and serve the soup warm.

Creamy Asparagus Soup

Time: 50 minutes
Servings: 4-6

Ingredients:

2 tablespoons olive oil
1 shallot, chopped
1 garlic clove, chopped
1 pound fresh asparagus, trimmed
½ teaspoon dried marjoram

3 cups chicken stock
1 cup water
Salt and pepper to taste
½ cup heavy cream

Directions:

1. Heat the oil in a soup pot and stir in the shallot and garlic.
2. Sauté for 2 minutes then add the asparagus, marjoram, stock, water, salt and pepper.
3. Cook for 30 minutes on low to medium flame.
4. Puree the soup with an immersion blender and pass it through a fine sieve for a smoother texture.
5. Stir in the cream and serve the soup warm.

Vegetable Soup with Cheese Topping

Time: 1¼ hours
Servings: 6-8

Ingredients:

2 tablespoons vegetable oil
1 red onion, chopped
1 zucchini, diced
1 carrot, diced
1 parsnip, diced
1 can fire roasted tomatoes
2 cups vegetable stock

3 cups water
½ teaspoon red pepper powder
½ teaspoon cumin seeds
Salt and pepper to taste
1 cup grated maturated cheese of your choice for serving

Directions:

1. Heat the oil in a soup pot and stir in the onion.
2. Sauté for 2 minutes then add the zucchini, carrot, parsnip, tomatoes, stock, water and spices.
3. Add salt and pepper to taste and cook the soup over medium flame for 20-30 minutes.
4. Serve the soup warm, topped with cheese.

Butternut Squash Soup

Time: 50 minutes
Servings: 4-6

Ingredients:

2 tablespoons olive oil
1 garlic clove, chopped
1 celery stalk, sliced
1 carrot, sliced
½ red pepper, seeded and chopped
½ teaspoon cumin seeds
3 cups butternut squash cubes
4 cups water
Salt and pepper to taste

Directions:

1. Heat the oil in a soup pot and stir in the garlic.
2. Sauté for 30 seconds then add the celery, carrot, red pepper, cumin seeds, squash and water.
3. Season with salt and pepper and cook for 25 minutes.
4. Puree the soup with an immersion blender and serve the soup warm.

Classic Chicken Soup

Time: 1½ hours
Servings: 6-8

Ingredients:

1 whole chicken, cut into small pieces
2 carrots, sliced
1 parsnip, sliced
2 celery stalks, sliced
1 leek, sliced
1 onion, sliced
7 cups water
1 bay leaf
Salt and pepper to taste

Directions:

1. Combine all the ingredients in a soup pot.
2. Add salt and pepper to taste and cook the soup over low heat for 1 hour.
3. Serve the soup warm.

Creamy Mushroom Soup

Time: 50 minutes
Servings: 4-6

Ingredients:

2 tablespoons butter
1 tablespoon olive oil
1 shallot, chopped
1 garlic clove, minced
1½ pounds mushrooms, sliced
1 cup chicken stock
2 cups water
Salt and pepper to taste
½ cup heavy cream

Directions:

1. Heat the butter with olive oil in a soup pot and stir in the shallot and garlic.
2. Sauté for 2 minutes then stir in mushrooms.
3. Add the stock, water, salt and pepper and cook the soup on medium flame for 20 minutes.
4. Puree the soup with an immersion blender and stir in the cream.
5. Bring to a boil and remove from heat.
6. Serve the soup warm.

Chinese Chicken Soup

Time: 45 minutes
Servings: 4-6

Ingredients:

6 cups chicken stock
2 Portobello mushrooms, sliced
1 celery stalk, sliced
2 garlic cloves, chopped
1 teaspoon grated ginger
2 cups shredded chicken
2 bok choys, shredded
2 tablespoons soy sauce
3 green onions, chopped

Directions:

1. Combine the stock, mushrooms, celery, garlic and ginger in a soup pot.
2. Bring to a boil then stir in the chicken and bok choy.
3. Cook the soup for 15 minutes then add the soy sauce and remove from heat.
4. Serve the soup warm, topped with green onions.

Creamy Tomato Soup

Time: 45 minutes
Servings: 4-6

Ingredients:

2 tablespoons olive oil
1 teaspoon dried basil
2 garlic cloves, minced
1 shallot, chopped
6 large ripe tomatoes, peeled and cubed
4 cups vegetable stock
Salt and pepper to taste
2 tablespoons chopped parsley

Directions:

1. Heat the oil in a soup pot and stir in the basil, garlic and shallot.
2. Sauté for 2 minutes then stir in the tomatoes, stock, salt and pepper.
3. Cook on medium flame for 25 minutes.
4. Puree the soup with an immersion blender and pass it thorough a fine sieve for a smoother texture.
5. Serve the soup topped with chopped parsley.

Creamy Butternut Squash Soup

Time: 50 minutes
Servings: 4-6

Ingredients:

2 tablespoons butter
1 shallot, chopped
2 garlic cloves, chopped
4 cups butternut squash cubes
3 cups vegetable stock
1 cup water
Salt and pepper to taste
½ cup heavy cream
1 red pepper for serving

Directions:

1. Melt the butter in a soup pot and stir in the shallot and garlic.
2. Sauté for 2 minutes then stir in the butternut squash cubes.
3. Add the stock, water, salt and pepper and cook the soup for 25 minutes.
4. Remove from heat, stir in the cream and puree the soup with an immersion blender until smooth.
5. Serve the soup warm, topped with a few red pepper slices.

Vietnamese Beef Soup

Time: 45 minutes
Servings: 6-8

Ingredients:

6 cups beef stock
2 teaspoon grated ginger
1 tablespoon fish sauce
2 cups sliced mushrooms
4 beef steaks, grilled and sliced
4 Thai basil leaves, chopped
2 tablespoons soy sauce
1 bok choy, shredded
4 green onions, finely sliced
2 tablespoons chopped cilantro

Directions:

1. Combine the stock, ginger, fish sauce, mushrooms, beef, basil and soy sauce in a soup pot.
2. Bring to a boil and cook for 15 minutes.
3. Add the bok choy, green onions and cilantro and cook 5 additional minutes.
4. Serve the soup warm.

Roasted Tomato Soup

Time: 1½ hours
Servings: 4-6

Ingredients:

6 ripe tomatoes, halved
2 garlic cloves
2 red onions, sliced
3 tablespoons olive oil
1 teaspoon dried basil
4 cups vegetable stock
1 cup water
Salt and pepper to taste

Directions:

1. Combine the tomatoes, garlic, red onions, olive oil and basil in a baking tray lined with parchment paper.
2. Roast in the preheated oven at 375F for 40 minutes.
3. Transfer the tomatoes in a soup pot and add the stock and water.
4. Adjust the taste with salt and pepper and cook the soup for 15 minutes.
5. Puree the soup with an immersion blender then pass the soup through a fine sieve.
6. Serve the soup warm.

Classic Chicken Soup with Egg Noodles

Time: 2 hours
Servings: 6-8

Ingredients:

1 whole chicken, cut into smaller pieces
8 cups water
2 carrots, cut into sticks
1 celery stalk, coarsely sliced
1 shallot, left whole
½ teaspoon black pepper kernels
Salt to taste
4 eggs, beaten

Directions:

1. Combine the chicken, water, carrots, celery, shallot and black pepper kernels in a soup pot.
2. Add salt to taste and cook over low heat for 1½ hours.
3. Turn the heat on high and stir well into the soup to form a whirl.
4. Quickly pour the eggs into the whirls and mix. This will form the egg noodles.
5. Serve the soup warm.

Salads

Mediterranean Calamari Salad

Time: 40 minutes
Servings: 4-6

Ingredients:

1½ pounds calamari, cut into rings
1 red pepper, sliced
2 garlic cloves, minced
2 tablespoons olive oil
½ lemon, juiced
2 cucumbers, sliced
1 cup chopped cilantro
1 red onion, sliced

Directions:

1. Mix the calamari rings with red pepper, garlic, olive oil and lemon juice in a bowl.
2. Heat a grill pan over medium flame. Place the calamari rings on the hot grill and cook for 2-3 minutes on each side.
3. Transfer the grilled calamari into a bowl and stir in the cucumbers, cilantro and red onions.
4. Drizzle with additional lemon juice if needed and serve the salad warm.

Grilled Chicken Salad

Time: 20 minutes
Servings: 4-6

Ingredients:

2 tablespoons Dijon mustard
¼ cup mayonnaise
½ lemon, juiced
2 tablespoons chopped parsley
1 head lettuce, shredded
3 chicken fillets, grilled and cut into thin strips

Directions:

1. Mix the mustard, mayonnaise, lemon juice and parsley in a small bowl.
2. Combine the lettuce with the dressing and transfer it on a platter.
3. Top with grilled chicken and serve immediately.

Artichoke Salad

Time: 20 minutes
Servings: 2-4

Ingredients:

1 jar artichoke hearts, chopped
2 green onions, chopped
1 tablespoon chopped parsley
½ cup mayonnaise
¼ cup plain yogurt
Salt and pepper to taste

Directions:

1. Mix the artichokes with green onions, parsley, mayonnaise and yogurt.
2. Add salt and pepper to taste and mix well.
3. Serve the salad fresh.

Tomato and Lettuce Salad

Time: 20 minutes
Servings: 4-6

Ingredients:

1 head lettuce, shredded
1 cup cherry tomatoes, halved
3 green onions, sliced
1 teaspoon chopped mint
2 tablespoons olive oil
2 tablespoons balsamic vinegar
Salt and pepper to taste

Directions:

1. Combine all the ingredients in a salad bowl.
2. Mix gently and serve the salad as fresh as possible.

Anchovy Salad Sauce

Time: 15 minutes
Servings: 4-6

Ingredients:

½ cup mayonnaise
6 anchovy fillets
2 tablespoons lemon juice
2 garlic cloves
Salt and pepper to taste

Directions:

1. Combine all the ingredients in a mortar and mix well with a pestle until smooth.
2. Drizzle the dressing over the salad just before serving.

Tamarind Asian Salad

Time: 20 minutes
Servings: 4-6

Ingredients:

1 head lettuce, shredded
2 green onions, sliced
2 cucumbers, sliced
2 tablespoons tamarind paste
2 tablespoon hot water
1 teaspoon rice vinegar
½ teaspoon chili paste
½ teaspoon sesame oil
2 tablespoons soy sauce
2 tablespoons sesame seeds

Directions:

1. Combine the lettuce, green onions and cucumbers in a bowl.
2. In a smaller bowl, mix the tamarind paste with hot water then add the remaining ingredients to make the dressing.
3. Drizzle the dressing over the salad and sprinkle with sesame seeds before serving.

Asian Pork Salad

Time: 20 minutes
Servings: 4

Ingredients:

2 garlic cloves, chopped
1 tablespoon rice vinegar
2 tablespoons lemon juice
2 tablespoons soy sauce
1 bag baby greens
1 cucumber, finely sliced
4 pork chops, cooked and sliced
2 green onions, sliced

Directions:

1. Combine the garlic, rice vinegar, lemon juice and soy sauce in a small bowl.
2. Mix the baby greens with cucumber and pork chops in a salad bowl.
3. Drizzle in the dressing and mix gently.
4. Serve the salad fresh. Garnish with green onions.

Onion Salad

Time: 15 minutes
Servings: 2-4

Ingredients:

- 4 green onions, sliced
- 2 red onions, sliced
- 1 tablespoon soy sauce
- 2 tablespoons rice vinegar
- ½ teaspoon chili flakes
- ½ teaspoon grated ginger

Directions:

1. Combine the green onions and red onions in a salad bowl.
2. Mix the soy sauce, vinegar, chili flakes and ginger in a bowl then drizzle this dressing over the salad.
3. Serve the salad fresh.

Gravlax Fennel Salad

Time: 30 minutes
Servings: 2-4

Ingredients:

- 1 fennel bulb
- 4 oz. gravlax, finely sliced
- ½ cup coarsely chopped parsley
- ½ red pepper, finely sliced
- 1 orange, cut into segments

Directions:

1. Finely slice the fennel bulb and place it on a platter.
2. Top with gravlax, parsley, red pepper and orange slices and serve the salad fresh.

Tomato Cheese Salad

Time: 25 minutes
Servings: 2-4

Ingredients:

- 3 cups cherry tomatoes, halved
- ½ cup cubed feta cheese
- ½ cup Parmesan shavings
- ½ teaspoon dried basil
- ½ teaspoon dried oregano
- 2 tablespoons olive oil
- 1 tablespoon balsamic vinegar

Directions:

1. Combine all the ingredients in a bowl and mix gently.

2. Serve the salad as fresh as possible.

Egg and Cauliflower Salad

Time: 35 minutes
Servings: 4-6

Ingredients:

1 head cauliflower, cut into florets
6 hard-boiled eggs
1 celery stalk, sliced
1 tablespoon Dijon mustard
½ cup light mayonnaise
2 tablespoons lemon juice
Salt and pepper to taste

Directions:

1. Cook the cauliflower in a steamer for 15 minutes then coarsely chop it.
2. Place the cauliflower in a bowl then stir in the eggs, celery, mustard, mayonnaise and lemon juice.
3. Add salt and pepper to taste and serve the salad fresh.

Kale Miso Salad

Time: 25 minutes
Servings: 2-4

Ingredients:

2 tablespoons miso paste
¼ cup warm water
2 green onions, chopped
½ red pepper, sliced
1 teaspoon rice vinegar
½ teaspoon sesame oil
5 cups shredded kale

Directions:

1. Combine the miso paste, water, onions, red pepper, vinegar and sesame oil in a small bowl.
2. Drizzle this dressing over the kale and mix to evenly coat the kale.
3. Serve the salad fresh.

Green Olive Kale Salad

Time: 15 minutes
Servings: 2-4

Ingredients:

4 cups shredded kale
½ cup green olives
1 green onion, sliced
1 ripe tomato, sliced
2 radishes, sliced
½ lemon, juiced
2 tablespoons olive oil
Salt and pepper to taste

Directions:

1. Combine the kale, olives, green onion, tomato and radishes in a salad bowl.
2. Drizzle with lemon juice and olive oil then season with salt and pepper and serve the salad fresh.

Caesar Salad

Time: 35 minutes
Servings: 2-4

Ingredients:

1 head lettuce, shredded
½ cup mayonnaise
2 garlic cloves, minced
2 tablespoons lemon juice
2 anchovies, chopped
4 bacon slices, cooked until crisp and shredded

Directions:

1. Place the lettuce on a platter.
2. Mix the mayonnaise with garlic, lemon juice and anchovies.
3. Drizzle this dressing over the salad and top with crushed bacon slices.
4. Serve the salad fresh.

Spicy Vegetable Salad

Time: 25 minutes
Servings: 2-4

Ingredients:

4 celery stalks, sliced
4 red bell peppers, cored and sliced
2 cucumbers, sliced
2 red peppers, seeded and sliced
1 lime, juiced
1 tablespoon balsamic vinegar
Salt and pepper to taste

Directions:

1. Combine all the ingredients in a bowl.
2. Add salt and pepper to taste and serve the salad fresh.

Cress Salad with Sweet Chili Dressing

Time: 25 minutes
Servings: 4-6

Ingredients:

1 head lettuce, shredded
2 cups garden cress
1 cucumber, finely sliced
2 tablespoons rice vinegar
2 tablespoons lemon juice
1 teaspoon sweet mustard
1 chili, finely sliced
2 tablespoons olive oil
½ teaspoon sesame oil
1 tablespoon soy sauce

Directions:

1. Combine the lettuce, cress and cucumber in a salad bowl.
2. Mix the vinegar, lemon juice, mustard, chili, olive oil and sesame oil in a small bowl. Add the soy sauce as well.
3. Drizzle the dressing over the salad and serve immediately.

Main Dishes

Rosemary Salmon and Braised Broccoli

Time: 40 minutes
Servings: 4

Ingredients:

4 salmon fillets
Salt and pepper to taste
2 rosemary sprigs, chopped
4 lemon slices
1 pound broccoli, cut into florets
2 tablespoons olive oil

Directions:

1. Season the salmon fillets with salt and pepper and place them in a baking pan lined with baking paper.
2. Sprinkle them with chopped rosemary and a slice of lemon.
3. Scatter the broccoli into the pan and season it with salt and pepper then drizzle with olive oil.
4. Cook in the preheated oven at 350F for 25-30 minutes.
5. Serve the salmon and broccoli warm.

Tangy Scrambled Eggs

Time: 30 minutes
Servings: 2-4

Ingredients:

5 eggs, beaten
2 tablespoons whole milk
1 ripe tomato, diced
Salt and pepper to taste
1 tablespoon butter
2 tablespoons olive oil

Directions:

1. Mix the eggs with milk, tomato, salt and pepper in a bowl.
2. Heat the butter and oil in a heavy saucepan then stir in the egg mixture.
3. Cook, stirring all the time, until set.
4. Serve the scrambled eggs warm.

Fish Pockets with Sautéed Mushrooms

Time: 1 hour
Servings: 4

Ingredients:

4 fish fillets of your choice
Salt and pepper to taste
1 teaspoon dried rosemary
1 teaspoon dried thyme

2 tablespoons butter
1 tablespoon olive oil
1 pound mushrooms, sliced

Directions:

1. Season the fish fillets with salt and pepper to taste, as well as rosemary and thyme.
2. Heat the butter and oil in a skillet and place the fish into the hot skillet.
3. Fry the fish on both sides until golden brown.
4. Remove the fish from the skillet and stir in the mushrooms into the hot oil and butter.
5. Cook the mushrooms for 10 minutes, stirring often.
6. Season with salt and pepper and serve the fish topped with mushrooms.

Breakfast from the West

Time: 30 minutes
Servings: 4

Ingredients:

3 tablespoons olive oil
1 pound breakfast sausages, sliced
1 sweet potato, diced

5 eggs, beaten
Salt and pepper to taste

Directions:

1. Heat the oil in a skillet and stir in the sausages and sweet potato.
2. Sauté for 10 minutes then stir in the eggs and mix until cooked and set. Add salt and pepper to taste.
3. Serve the dish warm.

Grilled Chicken with Buffalo Ranch Sauce

Time: 40 minutes
Servings: 4

Ingredients:

Grilled chicken:

4 chicken breasts, cut in half lengthwise

Salt and pepper to taste
1 teaspoon Cajun seasoning
1 teaspoon chili powder
½ teaspoon garlic powder
Sauce:
¼ cup mayonnaise
1 teaspoon dried parsley
½ teaspoon garlic powder
¼ teaspoon onion powder
1 teaspoon dried dill
1 tablespoon chopped chives
Salt and pepper to taste
1 teaspoon hot Buffalo sauce

Directions:

1. For the grilled chicken, season the chicken with salt, pepper, Cajun seasoning, chili powder and garlic powder.
2. Heat a grill pan over medium to high flame and place the chicken on the grill.
3. Cook on each side for 5-7 minutes.
4. To make the sauce, mix all the ingredients in a bowl.
5. Serve the warm grilled chicken topped with sauce.

Sausage and Pork Bake

Time: 1½ hours
Servings: 6-8

Ingredients:

1½ pounds pork shoulder
4 smoked sausages, sliced
2 Chorizo links, sliced
2 tablespoons vegetable oil
1 cup tomato sauce

Directions:

1. Combine all the ingredients in a deep dish baking pan.
2. Cook in the preheated oven at 350F for 1 hour.
3. Stir into the bake from time to time to ensure and even baking.
4. Serve the pork bake warm.

Egg Zucchini Casserole

Time: 55 minutes
Servings: 6-8

Ingredients:

4 eggs, beaten
1 cup sour cream

1½ cups milk
2 tablespoons coconut flour
1 teaspoon dried dill

Salt and pepper to taste
6 young zucchinis, sliced

Directions:

1. Mix the eggs, sour cream, milk, coconut flour, dill, salt and pepper in a bowl.
2. Layer the zucchinis in a deep dish baking pan then pour the egg mixture over the zucchinis.
3. Cook in the preheated oven at 350F for 40 minutes.
4. Let the zucchinis cool down before serving.

Bacon Wrapped Duck Breasts

Time: 40 minutes
Servings: 4

Ingredients:

4 duck breasts, skin off
Salt and pepper to taste

2 tablespoons olive oil
8 bacon slices

Directions:

1. Season he duck breasts with salt and pepper.
2. Heat the oil in a skillet then place the duck breasts into the hot oil and fry on all sides until golden brown.
3. Wrap the duck breasts in bacon slices and place them all in a baking tray.
4. Cook in the preheated oven at 375F for 20 minutes.
5. Serve the duck breasts warm.

Bacon Wrapped Meatloaf

Time: 1¼ hours
Servings: 8-10

Ingredients:

2 pounds ground pork
1 carrot, grated
2 tablespoons Dijon mustard
2 eggs
½ cup almond flour

1 teaspoon Worcestershire sauce
2 tablespoons chopped parsley
Salt and pepper to taste
8 bacon slices

Directions:

1. Mix the pork, carrot, mustard, eggs, almond flour, Worcestershire sauce and parsley in a bowl.
2. Season with salt and pepper then spoon the mixture into a loaf pan.
3. Top with bacon slices and cook in the preheated oven at 350F for 40-45 minutes or until fragrant and golden brown.
4. Let the mixture cool down before slicing and serving.

Onion and Sour Cream Pork Chops

Time: 1 hour
Servings: 4

Ingredients:

2 tablespoons olive oil
4 pork chops
2 sweet onions, sliced
1 cup sour cream
½ cup whole milk
Salt and pepper to taste

Directions:

1. Heat the olive oil in a skillet.
2. Place the pork chops in the hot oil and fry on both sides until golden brown.
3. Remove the pork chops from the skillet and stir the onion into the fat left in the pan.
4. Sauté for 5 minutes then place the pork chops back into the pan.
5. Mix the sour cream with milk in a bowl then pour it over the pork chops.
6. Season with salt and pepper and cook on medium flame for 10 minutes.
7. Serve the dish warm.

Cranberry Muscadine Pork Roast

Time: 2¼ hours
Servings: 6-8

Ingredients:

1 cup cranberry sauce
½ cup muscadine wine
Salt and pepper to taste
2½ pounds pork shoulder
1 cup vegetable stock

Directions:

1. Mix the cranberry sauce and wine in a bowl. Add salt and pepper to taste.
2. Spread the mixture over the pork shoulder then place the pork in a deep dish baking pan.
3. Pour in the stock and cook in the preheated oven at 350F for 1¾ hours.
4. Serve the pork roast warm.

Vegetable Medley

Time: 1 hour
Servings: 6-8

Ingredients:

2 tablespoons olive oil
2 zucchinis, sliced
2 yellow squashes, sliced
2 ripe tomatoes, sliced

1 teaspoon dried oregano
Salt and pepper to taste
2 tablespoons chopped parsley

Directions:

1. Heat the olive oil in a skillet and stir in the zucchinis, yellow squashes, tomatoes and dried oregano.
2. Season with salt and pepper and cook over medium flame for 15-20 minutes, stirring often.
3. Serve the veggie medley with freshly chopped parsley.

Cheesy Squash Casserole

Time: 1 hour
Servings: 4-6

Ingredients:

4 young yellow squashes, sliced
2 Vidalia onions, sliced
2 tomatoes, sliced
¼ cup butter, melted
Salt and pepper to taste
1 cup grated Romano cheese
1 cup shredded mozzarella

365 Days of Low Carb Recipes

Directions:

1. Mix the yellow squashes with onions and tomatoes in a deep dish baking pan.
2. Drizzle with melted butter then season with salt and pepper.
3. Top with Romano cheese and mozzarella and cook in the preheated oven at 350F for 40 minutes.
4. Serve the casserole warm.

Indian Style Tofu

Time: 30 minutes
Servings: 4

Ingredients:

1 teaspoon smoked paprika
1 teaspoon curry powder
½ teaspoon cumin powder
½ teaspoon turmeric powder
3 tablespoons olive oil
¼ cup low fat yogurt
¼ teaspoon garlic powder
4 thick slices firm tofu

Directions:

1. Mix the paprika, curry powder, cumin powder, turmeric, olive oil, yogurt and garlic powder in a bowl.
2. Brush the tofu slices with this mixture.
3. Heat a grill pan over medium flame.
4. Place the tofu over the grill and cook on both sides until golden brown.
5. Serve the tofu warm.

Sicilian Chicken

Time: 1¼ hours
Servings: 6-8

Ingredients:

½ cup green olives, halved
4 ripe tomatoes, cubed
1 teaspoon capers, chopped
½ teaspoon red pepper flakes
2 tablespoons olive oil
Salt and pepper to taste
1 whole chicken, cut into smaller pieces

Directions:

1. Mix the green olives, tomatoes, capers, red pepper flakes and olive oil in a deep dish baking pan.
2. Season with salt and pepper the chicken and place it over the veggies.
3. Cook in the preheated oven at 350F for 1 hour.
4. Serve the chicken warm.

White Fish with Tomato Salsa

Time: 50 minutes
Servings: 6

Ingredients:

6 white fish fillets of your choice
Salt and pepper to taste
3 tablespoons olive oil
3 ripe tomatoes, diced
1 green onion, chopped
¼ cup chopped cilantro
1 red pepper, chopped
1 lime, juiced

Directions:

1. Season the fish with salt and pepper and place the fillets on a baking sheet.
2. Drizzle with olive oil and cook in the preheated oven at 400F for 20 minutes.
3. For the salsa, mix the tomatoes with green onion, cilantro, red pepper and lime juice in a bowl.
4. Adjust the taste with salt and pepper.
5. Serve the cooked fish fillets with fresh salsa.

Chicken Paprikash

Time: 1 hour
Servings: 6

Ingredients:

6 chicken thighs
1 teaspoon sweet paprika
1 teaspoon hot paprika
Salt and pepper to taste
3 tablespoons olive oil
1 shallot, chopped
2 cups water

1 thyme sprig
½ cup milk
1 tablespoon cornstarch

Directions:

1. Sprinkle the chicken thighs with paprika, salt and pepper.
2. Heat the oil in a heavy saucepan and place the chicken in.
3. Cook the chicken on all sides until golden brown then add the shallot, water and thyme.
4. Cook over medium to low flame for 30 minutes.
5. Mix the milk with cornstarch and pour the mixture into the saucepan.
6. Cook just until it begins to thicken and serve the paprikash warm.

Tofu au Vin

Time: 1 hour
Servings: 6-8

Ingredients:

3 tablespoons olive oil
6 slices tofu, cubed
2 tablespoons tomato paste
2 garlic cloves, minced
1 carrot, sliced
1 cup pearl onions
1 pound mushrooms, sliced
1 fresh thyme sprig
2 cups water
1 cup vegetable stock
½ cup red wine
Salt and pepper to taste

Directions:

1. Heat the oil in a heavy saucepan and stir in the tofu cubes.
2. Cook on all sides until golden brown and crusty then stir in the tomato paste and garlic and sauté just 1 additional minute.
3. Stir in the remaining ingredients and adjust the taste with salt and pepper.
4. Cook the dish on medium flame for 30 minutes.
5. Serve warm.

Indian Spiced Chicken Stew

Time: 1¼ hours
Servings: 6-8

Ingredients:

- 3 tablespoons vegetable oil
- 1 whole chicken, cut into smaller pieces
- 1 teaspoon cumin seeds
- ½ teaspoon coriander seeds
- 1 teaspoon turmeric powder
- ½ teaspoon curry powder
- ½ teaspoon red pepper powder
- 1 sweet onion, chopped
- 2 garlic cloves, minced
- 1 cup diced tomatoes
- 1 pound asparagus, cut into smaller pieces
- 1½ cups water
- ½ cup coconut milk
- Salt and pepper to taste

Directions:

1. Heat the oil in a large heavy pot and stir in the chicken.
2. Cook on all sides until golden brown.
3. Stir in the cumin seeds, coriander seeds, turmeric powder, curry powder, red pepper powder, onions and garlic and sauté for 3 minutes, stirring often.
4. Add the tomatoes, asparagus, water and coconut milk, as well as salt and pepper and cook on medium flame for 30 minutes.
5. Serve the dish warm, topped with freshly chopped herbs.

Cheese Stuffed Chicken Breasts

Time: 1 hour
Servings: 4

Ingredients:

- 4 oz. mozzarella cheese
- 2 oz. grated Cheddar
- ½ teaspoon dried tarragon
- Salt and pepper to taste
- 4 chicken breasts
- 1 cup chicken stock
- 1 bay leaf

Directions:

1. Mix the mozzarella, Cheddar, tarragon, salt and pepper in a bowl.
2. Cut a small pocket into each chicken breast and stuff them all with the cheese mixture.
3. Place the chicken breasts in a deep dish baking pan and add the stock and bay leaf, as well as salt and pepper if needed.
4. Cook in the preheated oven at 375F for 35-40 minutes.
5. Serve the chicken warm with your favorite side dish or simple as it is.

Cheesy Turkey Meatballs

Time: 1¼ hours
Servings: 6-8

Ingredients:

2 pounds ground turkey
1 shallot, finely chopped
2 tablespoons chopped cilantro
½ teaspoon cumin powder
2 garlic cloves, minced
4 sun-dried tomatoes, finely chopped
1 egg
1 green onion, chopped
Salt and pepper to taste
6 oz. mozzarella, cut into small cubes

Directions:

1. Mix the turkey meat with shallot, cilantro, cumin powder, garlic, sun-dried tomatoes, egg and green onion in a bowl.
2. Add salt and pepper to taste then form small meatballs.
3. Flatten each meatball and place a mozzarella cube in the center. Wrap the edges around the cheese and shape into a ball again.
4. Place the meatballs on a baking tray lined with parchment paper.
5. Bake in the preheated oven at 350F for 25-30 minutes.
6. Serve the meatballs warm.

Turkey Meatballs in Tomato Sauce

Time: 1¼ hours
Servings: 6-8

Ingredients:

2 pounds ground turkey
2 garlic cloves, minced
1 sweet onion, chopped
1 egg
Salt and pepper to taste
2 tablespoons olive oil
1 shallot, chopped
1 can diced tomatoes
1 cup tomato sauce
1 bay leaf
1 thyme sprig
¼ cup white wine

Directions:

1. Mix the turkey with garlic, sweet onion and egg in a bowl.
2. Season with salt and pepper and form small meatballs.
3. Heat the olive oil in a skillet and stir in the shallot. Sauté for 2 minutes.

4. Add the tomatoes, tomato sauce, bay leaf, thyme and white wine and bring the sauce to a boil.
5. Lower the heat and place the meatballs into the hot sauce.
6. Cover with a lid and cook for 20-30 minutes.
7. Serve the meatballs warm, topped with plenty of sauce.

Cranberry Roasted Chicken

Time: 2 hours
Servings: 6-8

Ingredients:

1 cup cranberry sauce
1 teaspoon red pepper flakes
1 teaspoon cumin seeds
1 teaspoon Worcestershire sauce
2 tablespoons Dijon mustard
1 teaspoon salt
1 whole chicken

Directions:

1. Mix the cranberry sauce with the rest of the ingredients.
2. Place the chicken in a baking pan and spread the cranberry mixture over the chicken.
3. Cook in the preheated oven at 330F for 1 hour.
4. Turn the heat on high and cook for 30 additional minutes.
5. Serve the chicken warm, simple or with your favorite side dish.

Steak with Mushroom Sauce

Time: 1 hour
Servings: 4

Ingredients:

2 tablespoons olive oil
1 garlic clove, minced
½ pound mushrooms, chopped
½ teaspoon dried sage
¼ cup sherry
½ cup beef stock
½ cup heavy cream
4 beef steaks
Salt and pepper to taste

Directions:

1. Heat the oil in a skillet and stir in in the garlic.
2. Sauté for 30 seconds then add the mushrooms. Cook for 5-8 minutes then stir in the sage, sherry, stock and cream.
3. Lower the heat and cook the sauce for 10 minutes.
4. Season the steaks with salt and pepper.
5. Heat a grill pan over medium to high flame and place the steaks on the grill.
6. Cook them on each side for 5-6 minutes.
7. Serve the steaks topped with sherry and mushroom sauce.

Steak and Spinach Salad

Time: 45 minutes
Servings: 4

Ingredients:

4 steaks
Salt and pepper to taste
1 pound fresh baby spinach
2 tablespoons Dijon mustard
½ lemon, juiced
1 tablespoon balsamic vinegar
3 tablespoons olive oil

Directions:

1. Season the steaks with salt and pepper. Heat a grill pan over medium to high flame and place the steaks on the grill.
2. Cook the meat on each side for 5-7 minutes.
3. Place the spinach on a platter.
4. Make the dressing by mixing the mustard with lemon juice, balsamic vinegar and olive oil.
5. Drizzle the dressing over the spinach.
6. Cut the steaks into thin slices and place them on top of the salad.
7. Serve right away!

Chicken Cordon Bleu

Time: 1¼ hours
Servings: 6

Ingredients:

6 chicken fillets
12 bacon slices

12 sticks mozzarella cheese
Salt and pepper to taste
1 teaspoon dried basil

2 eggs, beaten
1 cup almond meal

Directions:

1. Lay the chicken fillets flat on your working surface.
2. Place 2 bacon slices on each chicken fillet then place 1 mozzarella stick on one side of the fillet and roll it tightly into the chicken.
3. Secure the ends of the cordon bleu with toothpicks if needed.
4. Season with salt, pepper and basil.
5. Roll the rolls though eggs and then through almond meal.
6. Place the rolls on a baking tray lined with baking paper.
7. Cook in the preheated oven at 475F for 20-30 minutes or until golden brown.
8. Serve the cordon bleu warm.

Pork Chops with Creamy Sauce

Time: 1 hour
Servings: 4

Ingredients:

2 tablespoons olive oil
4 pork chops, bone in
Salt and pepper to taste
½ cup water
1 shallot, chopped

1 cup sour cream
½ cup milk
1 pinch nutmeg
1 bay leaf

Directions:

1. Heat the oil in a skillet and place the pork chops in the hot skillet. Sprinkle with salt and pepper.
2. Cook on both sides until golden brown then add the water and cook until it evaporates.
3. Stir in the shallot and sauté for 2 minutes then add the sour cream, milk, nutmeg and bay leaf.
4. Reduce the heat on low and cook 10 minutes.
5. Serve the dish warm.

Ham Stuffed Pork Tenderloin

Time: 1½ hours
Servings: 6-8

Ingredients:

2-pound piece of pork tenderloin
Salt and pepper to taste
½ cup grated Parmesan
6 sage leaves
8 slices ham
1 cup chicken stock
1 rosemary sprig

Directions:

1. Cut the pork tenderloin on its fiber, carefully, to obtain a sheet of meat.
2. Season with salt and pepper then sprinkle with parmesan.
3. Top with sage leaves and ham slices then roll the tenderloin tightly.
4. Secure the ends with toothpicks and place the roll into a baking pan.
5. Add the stock and rosemary and cook in the preheated oven at 350F for 1 hour.
6. Serve the tenderloin warm, simple or with your favorite side dish.

Mustard Glazed Salmon

Time: 35 minutes
Servings: 4

Ingredients:

2 tablespoons Dijon mustard
2 tablespoons sweet mustard
2 tablespoons lemon juice
2 tablespoons olive oil
1 teaspoon dried sage
½ teaspoon salt
1 pinch chili flakes
4 salmon fillets

Directions:

1. Combine the mustard, lemon juice, olive oil, sage, salt and chili flakes in a bowl.
2. Place the salmon fillets in a baking tray lined with baking paper.
3. Brush the fish with the mustard mixture and cook in the preheated oven at 350F for 20 minutes.
4. Serve the salmon warm.

Chicken in Green Chile Sauce

Time: 1 hour
Servings: 4

Ingredients:

2 tablespoons olive oil
4 chicken breasts
2 garlic cloves, minced
2 green chiles, chopped
½ cup chopped cilantro
½ cup almond milk
1 cup chicken stock
Salt and pepper to taste

Directions:

1. Heat the oil in a skillet and place the chicken in the hot pan.
2. Cook the chicken on all sides until golden brown then remove it on a plate.
3. In the fat remaining in the pan, stir in the garlic, chiles and cilantro and sauté for 2 minutes.
4. Add the almond milk and stock and bring to a boil.
5. Place the chicken in the skillet as well and cook on low heat for 30 minutes. Add salt and pepper to taste.
6. Serve the chicken warm, topped with plenty of sauce.

Pork Chops in Marsala Sauce

Time: 45 minutes
Servings: 6

Ingredients:

6 pork chops, bone in
Salt and pepper to taste
6 bacon slices, chopped
1 leek, sliced
1 shallot, chopped
½ cup Marsala
½ cup chicken stock
½ cup heavy cream
2 tablespoons all-purpose flour

Directions:

1. Season the pork chops with salt and pepper.
2. Heat a skillet over medium flame and stir in the bacon.
3. Sauté for 5 minutes until crisp.
4. Add the leek and shallot and cook for 5 minutes until translucent.

5. Stir in the Marsala and stock and cook for 15 minutes.
6. Stir in the cream and cook 5 additional minutes. Thicken with flour as needed.
7. Remove from heat and serve the pork chops warm, topped with sauce.

Asian Style Steak

Time: 1 hour
Servings: 4

Ingredients:

2 green onions, chopped
¼ cup light soy sauce
1 teaspoon grated ginger
½ teaspoon red pepper flakes
½ teaspoon sesame oil
4 beef steaks

Directions:

1. Mix the onions, soy sauce, ginger, red pepper flakes and sesame oil in a bowl.
2. Place the steaks into the bowl as well and coat them well. Let them marinate for 30 minutes.
3. Heat a grill pan over medium to high flame and place the steaks on the hot grill.
4. Cook on both sides for 5-7 minutes and serve the steaks warm.

Garlicky Roasted Chicken

Time: 2 hours
Servings: 6-8

Ingredients:

6 garlic cloves, minced
1 teaspoon smoked paprika
½ teaspoon sweet paprika
½ teaspoon onion powder
1 teaspoon dried herbs of your choice
1 teaspoon salt
2 tablespoons olive oil
1 whole chicken

Directions:

1. Mix the garlic with paprika, onion powder, dried herbs, salt and olive oil in a small bowl.
2. Spread this mixture all over the chicken, rubbing it well into the skin.
3. Place the chicken in a deep baking pan and cover with aluminum foil.
4. Cook in the preheated oven at 350F for 1 hour then remove the foil and cook 30 additional minutes.

5. Serve the chicken warm.

Braised Paprika Chicken

Time: 1½ hours
Servings: 6

Ingredients:

2 red onions, sliced
2 red bell peppers, cored and sliced
1 cup chicken stock
Salt and pepper to taste
6 chicken thighs
1½ teaspoons smoked paprika

Directions:

1. Mix the onions and bell peppers in a deep dish baking pan.
2. Add the stock, as well as salt and pepper.
3. Season the chicken thighs with salt, pepper and paprika and place them over the onions.
4. Cook in the preheated oven at 350F for 1 hour.
5. Serve the chicken warm, topped with the sauce formed in the pan.

Butter Chicken

Time: 1¼ hours
Servings: 4

Ingredients:

¼ cup butter, softened
1 teaspoon chopped rosemary
1 teaspoon dried basil
½ teaspoon salt
½ teaspoon ground black pepper
4 chicken breasts

Directions:

1. Mix the butter, rosemary, basil, salt and black pepper in a bowl.
2. Place the chicken breasts in a baking tray.
3. Top each chicken breast with a dollop of butter mixture and cook in the preheated oven at 350F for 1 hour.
4. Serve the chicken warm.

Herbed Beef

Time: 40 minutes
Servings: 4

Ingredients:

4 beef steaks
2 tablespoons olive oil
2 tablespoons chopped parsley
1 teaspoon chopped rosemary
1 tablespoon chopped cilantro
½ teaspoon ground black pepper
½ teaspoon salt

Directions:

1. Drizzle the steaks with olive oil.
2. Mix the parsley with rosemary, cilantro, black pepper and salt in a bowl then roll the steaks through the chopped herbs.
3. Heat a grill pan over medium to high flame and place the steaks on the grill.
4. Cook them on each side for 5-7 minutes and serve them warm.

Beef Stroganoff in the Slow Cooker

Time: 6¼ hours
Servings: 2-4

Ingredients:

1 pound beef meat, cubed
Salt and pepper to taste
1 tablespoon all-purpose flour
2 tablespoons olive oil
1 large onion, chopped
2 carrots, sliced
1 can condensed cream of mushroom soup
1 bay leaf

Directions:

1. Season the beef with salt and pepper and sprinkle it with flour.
2. Heat the oil in a skillet and stir in the meat.
3. Cook on all sides until golden brown then transfer the meat in your slow cooker.
4. Add the remaining ingredients, as well as salt and pepper to taste and cook on low settings for 6 hours.
5. Serve the beef stroganoff warm.

Beef Carrot Stew

Time: 2¼ hours
Servings: 6-8

Ingredients:

3 tablespoons olive oil
1½ pounds beef meat, cubed
1 red onion, sliced
4 carrots, sliced

1 can diced tomatoes
1 cup beef stock
1 bay leaf
Salt and pepper to taste

Directions:

1. Heat the oil in a heavy pot and stir in the meat.
2. Sauté for 5 minutes then stir in the onion, carrots, tomatoes, stock and bay leaf.
3. Season with salt and pepper to taste.
4. Cover the pot with a lid and cook on low heat for 2 hours.
5. Serve the stew warm.

Beef Curry Stew

Time: 2 hours
Servings: 4-6

Ingredients:

2 tablespoons olive oil
2 pounds beef meat, cubed
2 garlic cloves, minced
1 sweet onion, chopped
½ teaspoon grated ginger

1 jalapeño pepper, chopped
1 teaspoon curry powder
1 can diced tomatoes
1 cup beef stock
Salt and pepper to taste

Directions:

1. Heat the oil in a heavy pot and stir in the beef.
2. Cook for 5 minutes on all sides then stir in the garlic and onion.
3. Sauté for 5 additional minutes then add the remaining ingredients.
4. Season with salt and pepper then lower the heat and cook the stew for 1½ hours.
5. Serve the stew warm.

Slow Cooker Beef Roast

Time: 6½ hours
Servings: 4-6

Ingredients:

2 pounds beef roast
Salt and pepper to taste
1 teaspoon smoked paprika
½ teaspoon chili powder
1 can condensed cream of mushroom soup

Directions:

1. Season the beef with salt and pepper then sprinkle it with paprika and chili powder.
2. Place the beef roast in the crock pot and add the mushroom soup.
3. Cook on low settings for 6 hours.
4. Serve the beef roast warm.

Ketchup Meatballs

Time: 50 minutes
Servings: 6-8

Ingredients:

2 pounds ground chicken
1 green onion, chopped
2 garlic cloves, chopped
1 teaspoon dried Italian herbs
Salt and pepper to taste
2 cups ketchup
1 can diced tomatoes
½ cup chicken stock
1 bay leaf

Directions:

1. Mix the ground chicken with green onion, garlic, herbs, salt and pepper.
2. Wet your hands and form small meatballs. Place them all on a chopping board.
3. For the sauce, combine the ketchup with tomatoes, stock and bay leaf in a saucepan and heat.
4. Add salt and pepper to taste then place the meatballs in the hot sauce.
5. Cook over medium to low heat for 30 minutes and serve the dish warm.

No Bean Chili

Time: 1¼ hours
Servings: 6-8

Ingredients:

3 tablespoons olive oil
4 bacon slices, chopped
2 pounds ground beef
2 sweet onions, chopped
2 garlic cloves, minced
½ teaspoon grated ginger
2 cans diced tomatoes
½ cup beef stock
Salt and pepper to taste

Directions:

1. Heat the oil in a heavy pot and stir in the bacon.
2. Cook until crisp then add the ground beef and sauté for 10 minutes, stirring often.
3. Stir in the onions and garlic and cook 2 additional minutes then add the remaining ingredients and season with salt and pepper.
4. Cook on low settings for 50 minutes.
5. Serve the chili warm.

Grilled Steaks with Eggplants

Time: 45 minutes
Servings: 4

Ingredients:

4 beef steaks
Salt and pepper to taste
2 eggplants, peeled and sliced
3 tablespoons olive oil
2 tablespoons balsamic vinegar

Directions:

1. Season the steaks with salt and pepper then heat a grill pan over medium flame. Place the steaks on the grill and cook them on both sides for 5-7 minutes or until golden brown.
2. Season the eggplants with salt and pepper then brush each slice with olive oil.
3. Cook the eggplants on the grill as well just until softened then drizzle them with balsamic vinegar.
4. Serve the steaks with balsamic eggplant slices.

Beef and Portobello Stir-Fry

Time: 45 minutes
Servings: 4

Ingredients:

3 tablespoons vegetable oil
1 pound beef steaks, cut into thin strips
2 garlic cloves, chopped
½ teaspoon grated ginger
4 Portobello mushrooms, sliced
2 tablespoons soy sauce

Directions:

1. Heat the oil in a large wok.
2. Stir in the beef and cook for 5 minutes on high heat, stirring often.
3. Add the garlic, ginger and mushrooms and keep cooking for 10-15 minutes, stirring often, until most of the liquid has evaporated.
4. Add the soy sauce and serve the stir-fry warm.

Red Snapper with Lychee

Time: 40 minutes
Servings: 4

Ingredients:

4 red snapper fillets
Salt and pepper to taste
2 tablespoons olive oil
6 peeled lychees, sliced
¼ cup chopped coriander
1 lime, juiced

Directions:

1. Season the red snapper with salt and pepper.
2. Heat the oil in a skillet and place the fish fillets in the hot oil.
3. Cook on each side for 3-4 minutes then remove the fish on a plate.
4. In the oil left in the pan, stir in the lychees, coriander and lime juice.
5. Lower the heat and sauté for 5-7 minutes.
6. Serve the fish fillets topped with lychee sauce.

Fish Chili with Lemongrass

Time: 1 hour
Servings: 6

Ingredients:

2 tablespoons olive oil
1 teaspoon grated ginger
1 shallot, sliced
1 can diced tomatoes
1 cup vegetable stock
½ teaspoon chili flakes
¼ lemongrass stalk, crushed
6 fish fillets of your choice
Salt and pepper to taste

Directions:

1. Heat the oil in a heavy saucepan and stir in the ginger and shallot.
2. Sauté for 2 minutes then add the tomatoes, stock, chili flakes and lemongrass.
3. Bring to a boil then add the fish fillets.
4. Season with salt and pepper and cook on low heat for 30 minutes.
5. Serve the chili warm.

Thai Fish Cakes

Time: 45 minutes
Servings: 4-6

Ingredients:

1½ pounds white fish
2 green onions, chopped
½ red pepper, chopped
1 egg
Salt and pepper to taste
4 tablespoons vegetable oil for frying

Directions:

1. Place the fish in a food processor and pulse until ground.
2. Stir in the green onions, red pepper and egg, as well as salt and pepper and mix well.
3. Heat the oil in a skillet then drop spoonfuls of fish mixture into the hot oil.
4. Fry on both sides until golden brown and serve the fish cakes warm.

Lamb Korma

Time: 1 hour
Servings: 4-6

Ingredients:

1 pound lamb shoulder, cut in thins strips
1 teaspoon smoked paprika
1 teaspoon cumin seeds
½ teaspoon cinnamon powder
Salt and pepper to taste
3 tablespoons olive oil
2 onions, chopped
1 cup vegetable stock
Plain yogurt for serving

Directions:

1. Mix the meat strips with paprika, cumin seeds, cinnamon, salt and pepper in a bowl.
2. Heat the oil in a skillet and add the meat.
3. Cook for 5-8 minutes until slightly golden brown then add the onions and stock.
4. Lower the heat and cook for 20-25 minutes until the liquid has evaporated and the meat begins to fry.
5. Cook just until it begins to thicken and become golden and serve warm, topped with yogurt.

Almond Cream Sauce Chicken

Time: 50 minutes
Servings: 6

Ingredients:

1 cup almonds
1 cup almond milk
1 cup chicken stock
2 tablespoons olive oil
6 chicken thighs, skin removed
2 garlic cloves, minced
1 shallot, chopped
Salt and pepper to taste
1 bay leaf

Directions:

1. Mix the almonds, almond milk and stock in a blender and pulse until smooth.
2. Heat the oil in a skillet and stir in the chicken.
3. Cook on all sides until golden brown then add the garlic and shallot.
4. Pour in the almond mixture then add salt and pepper to taste.
5. Add the bay leaf, lower the heat and cook for 30 minutes.
6. Serve the chicken warm, topped with plenty of sauce.

Grilled Jumbo Prawns

Time: 35 minutes
Servings: 2-4

Ingredients:

1 red pepper, sliced
1 lime, juiced
4 tablespoons olive oil
1 pinch salt
¼ teaspoon cumin powder
2 tablespoons soy sauce
1 teaspoon fish sauce
2 pounds jumbo prawns

Directions:

1. Mix the red pepper, lime juice, olive oil, salt, cumin powder, soy sauce and fish sauce in a bowl.
2. Place the jumbo prawns on wooden skewers then brush the prawns with the sauce you made earlier.
3. Heat a grill pan over medium to high flame.
4. Place the skewers on the grill and cook on both sides until golden brown.
5. Serve the prawns warm.

Cheesy Baked Chicken

Time: 1¼ hours
Servings: 6

Ingredients:

1 cup almond meal
½ cup grated Parmesan
½ teaspoon ground black pepper
6 chicken thighs
2 eggs, beaten
6 slices mozzarella cheese

Directions:

1. Mix the almond meal, Parmesan and black pepper in a bowl.
2. Dip the chicken thighs in beaten egg then roll them through the almond meal mixture.
3. Place the chicken thighs on a baking tray lined with parchment paper and top each thigh with a slice of mozzarella.
4. Cook in the preheated oven at 350F for 50 minutes.
5. Serve the chicken warm.

Honey Glazed Chicken Thighs

Time: 1¼ hours
Servings: 6

Ingredients:

2 tablespoons honey
2 tablespoons Dijon mustard
½ teaspoon chili flakes
1 teaspoon salt
6 chicken thighs

Directions:

1. Mix the honey, mustard, chili flakes and salt in a bowl.
2. Brush the chicken thighs with this mixture and place them in a baking tray lined with parchment paper.
3. Cook in the preheated oven at 350F for 45 minutes.
4. Serve the chicken thighs warm, simple or with your favorite side dish.

Beef Ragu

Time: 1½ hours
Servings: 8-10

Ingredients:

3 tablespoons olive oil
2 pounds ground beef
2 red onions, finely chopped
4 garlic cloves, minced
2 cans diced tomatoes
2 cups tomato sauce
2 bay leaves
Salt and pepper to taste

Directions:

1. Heat the oil in a heavy saucepan.
2. Stir in the beef and cook for 10 minutes.
3. Add the onion and garlic and cook for 10 additional minutes.
4. Stir in the diced tomatoes, tomato sauce, bay leaves, salt and pepper to taste.
5. Lower the heat and cook the ragu for 1 hour.
6. Serve the ragu warm or freeze it into individual portions.

Sticky Roasted Chicken

Time: 2 hours
Servings: 6-8

Ingredients:

¼ cup Dijon mustard
2 tablespoons honey
2 tablespoons olive oil
1 teaspoon dried thyme

½ teaspoon cayenne pepper
1 teaspoon onion powder
1 teaspoon salt
1 whole chicken

Directions:

1. Mix the mustard, honey, olive oil thyme, cayenne pepper, onion powder and salt in a bowl.
2. Spread this mixture over the chicken then place the chicken in a baking tray.
3. Cook in the preheated oven at 350F for 1½ hours.
4. Serve the chicken warm, simple or with your favorite side dish.

Spicy Roasted Chicken

Time: 1¼ hours
Servings: 6

Ingredients:

1 teaspoon smoked paprika
½ teaspoon chili flakes
2 tablespoons Dijon mustard
1 teaspoon dried sage

1 teaspoon salt
½ cup chicken stock
6 chicken thighs

Directions:

1. Mix the paprika, chili flakes, mustard, sage and salt in a bowl.
2. Brush the chicken thighs with this mixture and place them all in a baking tray.
3. Add the stock and cook in the preheated oven at 350F for 1 hour.
4. Serve the thighs warm.

Succulent Roasted Chicken

Time: 2 hours
Servings: 6-8

365 Days of Low Carb Recipes

Ingredients:

½ cup butter, softened
1 teaspoon sweet paprika
1 teaspoon dried oregano
1 teaspoon dried basil
1 teaspoon salt
1 teaspoon dried sage
1 whole chicken
1 cup chicken stock

Directions:

1. Mix the butter, paprika, oregano, basil, salt and sage in a bowl.
2. Place the chicken in a baking tray then cover it with butter mixture.
3. Add the stock in the tray as well.
4. Cook in the preheated oven at 350F for 1½ hours.
5. Serve the chicken warm, simple or with your favorite side dish.

Caribbean Roasted Chicken

Time: 2 hours
Servings: 6-8

Ingredients:

2 tablespoons olive oil
¼ cup dark rum
1 teaspoon cayenne pepper
1 teaspoon grated ginger
¼ teaspoon cinnamon powder
1 teaspoon salt
1 whole chicken

Directions:

1. Mix the olive oil, rum, cayenne, ginger, cinnamon powder and salt in a small bowl.
2. Brush the chicken with this mixture and place it in a baking tray.
3. Cook in the preheated oven at 350F for 1½ hours.
4. Serve the chicken warm, simple or with your favorite side dish.

Vegetable Frittata

Time: 35 minutes
Servings: 4-6

Ingredients:

6 eggs, beaten
½ cup heavy cream
1 teaspoon dried Italian herbs
Salt and pepper to taste

1 zucchini, sliced
1 green onion, chopped

2 red bell peppers, cored and sliced
2 tablespoons butter

Directions:

1. Mix the eggs with cream, herbs, salt and pepper. Stir in the zucchini, green onion and bell peppers.
2. Melt the butter in a skillet then pour in the frittata mixture.
3. Lower the heat and cover the skillet with a lid.
4. Cook on one side until set on top then carefully flip the frittata over and cook it a few more minutes.
5. Serve the frittata warm.

Seafood Tomato Stew

Time: 1 hour
Servings: 4-6

Ingredients:

2 tablespoons olive oil
1 shallot, chopped
2 garlic cloves, chopped
1 can diced tomatoes
1 cup tomato sauce

½ teaspoon cayenne pepper
10 oz. fresh prawns, peeled and deveined
10 oz. fresh scallops, cleaned
10 oz. white fish fillets, cubed
2 tablespoons chopped cilantro

Directions:

1. Heat the oil in a skillet and stir in the shallot and garlic.
2. Sauté for 2 minutes then add the tomatoes and tomato sauce.
3. Add the cayenne pepper and bring the sauce to a boil.
4. Cook the sauce for 15 minutes on low heat then carefully stir in the prawns, scallops and fish fillets.
5. Cook for 15 additional minutes covered with a lid.
6. Serve the stew warm, topped with chopped cilantro.

Green Salsa Chicken

Time: 1¼ hours
Servings: 4

Ingredients:

1 jar green salsa
½ cup chopped cilantro
1 cup chicken stock
Salt and pepper to taste
4 chicken breasts

Directions:

1. Mix the green salsa, cilantro and stock in a deep baking pan.
2. Add salt and pepper to taste then place the chicken breasts on top of the salsa.
3. Cook in the preheated oven at 350F for 1 hour.
4. Serve the chicken warm, topped with salsa.

Green Turkey Chili

Time: 1 hour
Servings: 4-6

Ingredients:

2 tablespoons olive oil
1½ pounds turkey breast, cubed
1 sweet onion, chopped
2 garlic cloves, minced
1 jar green salsa
½ cup chopped cilantro
2 jalapeno peppers, chopped
1 cup chicken stock
Salt and pepper to taste

Directions:

1. Heat the oil in a skillet and stir in the turkey.
2. Cook on all sides until slightly golden brown then stir in the onion and garlic.
3. Sauté for 2 additional minutes then add the remaining ingredients.
4. Season with salt and pepper and cook the chili for 40 minutes on low heat.
5. Serve the chili warm.

Korean Style Chicken

Time: 1½ hours
Servings: 4

Ingredients:

2 tablespoons Splenda
1 teaspoon sesame oil
4 green onions, chopped
¼ cup soy sauce

½ red pepper, chopped

4 chicken breasts

Directions:

1. Combine the Splenda, sesame oil, green onions, soy sauce and red pepper in a bowl.
2. Add the chicken and marinate for 30 minutes.
3. Heat the grill over medium flame and place the chicken breasts on the grill.
4. Cook on each side for 10-15 minutes, flipping them over often.
5. Serve the chicken warm, simple or with your favorite side dish.

Queso Chicken

Time: 1¼ hours
Servings: 4

Ingredients:

4 chicken breasts
2 tablespoons taco seasoning
½ cup heavy cream

1 cup chicken stock
1 cup grated Cheddar

Directions:

1. Season the chicken with taco seasoning.
2. Mix the cream with stock in a deep dish baking pan.
3. Add the chicken and top with cheese.
4. Cook in the preheated oven at 350F for 40-50 minutes.
5. Serve the chicken warm.

Chicken Kabobs

Time: 1 hour
Servings: 2-4

Ingredients:

2 chicken breasts, cubed
2 red bell peppers, cored and coarsely chopped
1 cup pearl onions
1 cup button mushrooms
1 teaspoon Italian herbs

1 teaspoon salt
1 teaspoon smoked paprika

Directions:

1. Place the chicken, bell peppers, pearl onions and mushrooms on wooden skewers.
2. Season the kabobs with herbs, salt and paprika.
3. Heat a grill pan over medium flame then place the kabobs on the grill and cook them on each side for 5-6 minutes or until golden brown.
4. Serve the kabobs warm.

Almond Crusted Chicken

Time: 1¼ hours
Servings: 6

Ingredients:

6 chicken thighs
1½ teaspoons salt
1 teaspoon cayenne pepper

2 eggs, beaten
1 cup almond slices
3 tablespoons olive oil

Directions:

1. Season the chicken with salt and cayenne pepper.
2. Dip each chicken thigh into egg then roll it through almond slices.
3. Place all the thighs on a baking tray and drizzle with olive oil.
4. Cook in the preheated oven at 350F for 1 hour.
5. Serve the chicken warm, simple or with your favorite side dish.

Coconut Poached Salmon

Time: 45 minutes
Servings: 4

Ingredients:

1 cup coconut milk
2 cups vegetable stock
1 bay leaf
¼ lemongrass stalk, crushed

½ celery stalk, sliced
1 carrot, sliced
Salt and pepper to taste
4 salmon fillets

Directions:

1. Combine the coconut milk, stock, bay leaf, lemongrass, celery and carrot in a saucepan.

2. Add a pinch of salt and pepper and bring to a boil.
3. When the liquid is boiling, place the salmon fillets in and cover the saucepan with a lid.
4. Cook for 20 minutes and serve the fish warm.

Coconut Crusted Fish

Time: 45 minutes
Servings: 6

Ingredients:

1 cup shredded coconut
2 tablespoons coconut flour
1 teaspoon salt
½ teaspoon ground black pepper
¼ teaspoon smoked paprika
6 white fish fillets
4 tablespoons coconut oil for frying

Directions:

1. Mix the shredded coconut, coconut flour, salt, black pepper and paprika in a bowl.
2. Roll the white fish fillets through the coconut mixture.
3. Heat the oil in a large skillet and place the fish fillets in the hot oil.
4. Fry on each side for 4-5 minutes or until golden brown.
5. Serve the fish warm.

Almond Crusted Fish with Leeks

Time: 1 hour
Servings: 6

Ingredients:

2 tablespoons butter
4 leeks, sliced
½ cup almond flour
½ cup almond slices
1 teaspoon dried Italian herbs
1 teaspoon salt
6 white fish fillets
1 egg, beaten

Directions:

1. Heat the butter in a skillet and stir in the leeks. Sauté for 10 minutes then transfer the mixture in a deep dish baking pan.
2. Mix the almond flour, almond slices, herbs and salt in a bowl.
3. Dip the fish fillets in egg then coat them in the almond mixture.

4. Place them over the leeks and cook in the preheated oven at 350F for 30 minutes.
5. Serve the fish warm, topped with plenty of leeks.

Macadamia Crusted Lamb

Time: 1 hour
Servings: 6

Ingredients:

6 lamb cutlets
Salt and pepper to taste
2 tablespoons olive oil
¾ cup macadamia nuts, ground
2 tablespoons chopped rosemary

Directions:

1. Season the lamb with salt and pepper and drizzle the cutlets with olive oil.
2. Mix the macadamia nuts with rosemary then roll the lamb cutlets through the mixture.
3. Place them on a baking tray lined with parchment paper and cook in the preheated oven at 350F for 25 minutes.
4. Serve the lamb cutlets warm with your favorite side dish.

Artichoke Frittata

Time: 35 minutes
Servings: 6-8

Ingredients:

3 tablespoons olive oil
1 red onion, chopped
1 garlic clove, minced
6 artichoke hearts, chopped
6 eggs, beaten
Salt and pepper to taste

Directions:

1. Heat the oil in a skillet and stir in the onion and garlic.
2. Sauté for 2 minutes then add the artichoke hearts.
3. Sauté for 2 additional minutes then stir in the eggs. Add salt and pepper to taste.
4. Lower the heat and cook the frittata for 15 minutes.
5. Flip it over carefully and cook a few more minutes until golden brown.
6. Serve the frittata warm.

Asian Style Patties

Time: 45 minutes
Servings: 4-6

Ingredients:

1½ pounds ground pork
1 carrot, grated
2 garlic cloves, minced
1 red onion, finely chopped
½ teaspoon sesame oil

2 tablespoons soy sauce
¼ teaspoon chili flakes
¼ cup sesame seeds
Oil for frying

Directions:

1. Mix the pork, carrot, garlic, red onion, sesame oil, soy sauce and chili flakes in a bowl.
2. Form small patties and roll each one of them through sesame seeds.
3. Heat a few tablespoons of oil in a skillet and place the pork patties in the hot oil.
4. Fry on each side for 3-4 minutes or until golden brown.
5. Remove them on paper towels and serve them warm or chilled.

Asian Chicken Thighs

Time: 1 hour
Servings: 6

Ingredients:

6 chicken thighs
1 tablespoon honey
¼ cup soy sauce
1 teaspoon grated ginger

½ teaspoon chili flakes
2 garlic cloves, minced
1 teaspoon rice vinegar

Directions:

1. Combine all the ingredients in a bowl and toss around to mix well.
2. Place the chicken thighs in a baking tray and cook in the preheated oven at 350F for 45 minutes.
3. Serve the chicken thighs warm, simple or with your favorite side dish.

Mediterranean Style Salmon Fillets

Time: 45 minutes
Servings: 6

Ingredients:

4 ripe tomatoes, sliced
½ cup black olives, pitted
4 basil leaves, chopped
½ cup crumbled feta cheese
½ cup almond meal
¼ cup chopped parsley
6 salmon fillets
Salt and pepper to taste

Directions:

1. Combine the tomatoes, black olives and basil in a deep dish baking pan.
2. Mix the feta with almond meal and parsley in a bowl.
3. Place the salmon fillets in the baking pan and top with the almond mixture. Add salt and pepper to taste.
4. Cook in the preheated oven at 350F for 25 minutes or until the top is golden brown and crusty.
5. Serve the salmon warm.

Balsamic Glazed Lamb Cutlets

Time: 1 hour
Servings: 6

Ingredients:

¼ cup balsamic vinegar
2 garlic cloves, minced
Salt and pepper to taste
6 lamb cutlets

Directions:

1. Mix the balsamic vinegar with garlic, salt and pepper.
2. Brush the lamb cutlets with the balsamic vinegar and let them marinate for 15 minutes.
3. Heat a grill pan over medium flame and place the lamb on the grill.
4. Cook on each side for 5-6 minutes and serve the cutlets warm, simple or with your favorite side dish.

BBQ Chicken Burgers

Time: 1 hour
Servings: 6

Ingredients:

1½ pounds ground chicken
1 green pepper, chopped
¼ cup BBQ sauce
1 egg
2 green onions, chopped
2 garlic cloves, minced
¼ cup chopped cilantro
Salt and pepper to taste

Directions:

1. Combine all the ingredients in a bowl and mix well.
2. Heat a grill pan over medium flame.
3. Form medium size burgers and place them on the grill.
4. Cook on each side for 4-5 minutes and serve the burgers warm with your favorite toppings.

BBQ Fish

Time: 35 minutes
Servings: 4

Ingredients:

4 salmon fillets
1 cup BBQ sauce
2 green onions, chopped
2 garlic cloves, minced
Salt and pepper to taste

Directions:

1. Combine all the ingredients in a deep dish baking pan.
2. Season with salt and pepper and cook in the preheated oven at 350F for 20 minutes.
3. Serve the fish warm.

Greek Omelet

Time: 25 minutes
Servings: 4-6

Ingredients:

5 eggs, beaten
2 tomatoes, diced
¼ cup crumbled feta
2 tablespoons chopped parsley
½ teaspoon dried oregano
3 tablespoons olive oil

Directions:

1. Mix the eggs, tomatoes, feta, parsley and oregano in a bowl.
2. Heat the oil in a skillet and stir in the egg mixture.
3. Cook the omelet on each side for 3-4 minutes or until golden brown.
4. Serve the omelet warm.

Seafood Curry

Time: 45 minutes
Servings: 4-6

Ingredients:

2 tablespoons butter
1 sweet onion, chopped
1 teaspoon turmeric powder
1 tablespoon red chili paste
2 tablespoons red curry paste
1 can diced tomatoes
Salt and pepper to taste
½ pound fresh prawns, peeled and deveined
4 salmon fillets, cubed
¼ pound mussels, cleaned
¼ cup chopped cilantro

Directions:

1. Melt the butter in a skillet and stir in the sweet onion.
2. Sauté for 2 minutes then add the turmeric powder, chili paste, curry paste and tomatoes.
3. Adjust the taste with salt and pepper and cook for 10 minutes.
4. Add the seafood, season with salt and pepper and cover the skillet with a lid.
5. Cook for 10 minutes then remove from heat and sprinkle with chopped cilantro to serve.

Tomato Basil Haddock

Time: 40 minutes
Servings: 4

Ingredients:

2 tablespoons olive oil
2 garlic cloves, minced
1 teaspoon dried oregano
1 teaspoon dried basil
1 can diced tomatoes
1 cup tomato sauce
Salt and pepper to taste
4 haddock fillets

Directions:

1. Heat the olive oil and stir in the garlic. Sauté for 30 seconds then stir in the oregano, basil, tomatoes and tomato sauce.
2. Add salt and pepper to taste and bring the sauce to a boil.
3. Cook for 10 minutes then place the haddock fillets in the hot sauce.
4. Cook 15 additional minutes and serve the fish warm, topped with plenty of sauce.

Parmesan Eggplants

Time: 45 minutes
Servings: 2-4

Ingredients:

½ cup almond meal
½ cup grated Parmesan
½ teaspoon dried basil
1 pinch salt
2 eggplants, peeled and sliced
2 eggs, beaten

Directions:

1. Mix the almond meal, Parmesan, basil and salt in a bowl.
2. Dip the eggplant slices in egg then roll each slice through the Parmesan mixture.
3. Place the eggplants on a baking tray lined with parchment paper.
4. Cook in the preheated oven at 350F for 30 minutes.
5. Serve the eggplants warm.

Tomato and Zucchini Stew

Time: 40 minutes
Servings: 4-6

Ingredients:

3 zucchinis, sliced
4 ripe tomatoes, sliced
1 teaspoon dried basil
Salt and pepper to taste

½ cup grated Parmesan

Directions:

1. Combine the zucchinis, tomatoes, basil, salt and pepper in a small deep dish baking pan.
2. Top with grated Parmesan and cook in the preheated oven at 350F for 25 minutes.
3. Serve the stew warm.

Cream Cheese Chicken

Time: 1 hour
Servings: 4

Ingredients:

2 tablespoons butter
4 chicken breasts
1 cup cream cheese
½ teaspoon dried basil
½ teaspoon dried oregano
1½ cups chicken stock
Salt and pepper to taste
1 cup shredded mozzarella

Directions:

1. Melt the butter in a skillet that can go in the oven.
2. Place the chicken breasts in the hot butter and cook on each side until golden brown.
3. Mix the cream cheese, basil, oregano, stock, salt and pepper in a bowl and pour this mixture over the chicken.
4. Top with shredded mozzarella and cook in the preheated oven at 350F for 25 minutes.
5. Serve the chicken warm, topped with plenty of sauce.

Poached Tilapia with Mayonnaise Sauce

Time: 40 minutes
Servings: 6

Ingredients:

4 cups water
½ lemon, sliced
1 bay leaf
Salt and pepper to taste
6 tilapia fillets
¼ cup mayonnaise
¼ cup plain yogurt
2 garlic cloves, minced

1 tablespoon chopped dill

Directions:

1. Combine the water, lemon slices, bay leaf, salt and pepper in a saucepan.
2. Bring the water to a boil then place the tilapia fillets in the hot water.
3. Cook for 15 minutes then carefully drain the tilapia.
4. For the mayonnaise sauce, combine the mayonnaise with yogurt, garlic and dill and drizzle this sauce over the tilapia fillets before serving.

Herb Crusted Salmon

Time: 45 minutes
Servings: 4

Ingredients:

1 cup chopped parsley
½ cup almond flour
1 teaspoon dried basil
¼ teaspoon chili flakes
1 teaspoon salt
4 salmon fillets

Directions:

1. Mix the parsley, almond flour, basil, chili flakes and salt in a bowl.
2. Place the salmon fillets in a baking tray.
3. Top each fish fillets with a few spoonfuls of parsley mixture and cook in the preheated oven at 350F for 20-25 minutes.
4. Serve the salmon fillets warm.

Puff Pastry Wrapped Salmon

Time: 1 hour
Servings: 4-6

Ingredients:

1 puff pastry sheet
2 tablespoons Dijon mustard
2 pound piece of salmon
Salt and pepper to taste

Directions:

1. Lay the puff pastry flat on your working surface.
2. Brush the puff pastry with mustard then place the salmon in the center.

3. Wrap the edges of the puff pastry over the fish and seal well.
4. Cook in the preheated oven at 375F for 20-30 minutes or until well puffed up and golden brown.
5. Serve the salmon warm.

Baby Spinach Omelet

Time: 25 minutes
Servings: 2-4

Ingredients:

2 tablespoons olive oil
2 cups baby spinach
¼ teaspoon onion powder

5 eggs, beaten
½ cup grated Parmesan

Directions:

1. Heat the oil in a skillet and stir in the baby spinach and onion powder.
2. Cook for 5 minutes until softened then stir in the eggs and cheese.
3. Cook a few additional minutes until set and serve the omelet warm.

Rotisserie Chicken

Time: 2 hours
Servings: 6-8

Ingredients:

¼ cup melted butter
1 teaspoon smoked paprika
1 teaspoon Cajun seasoning

1 teaspoon salt
1 whole chicken

Directions:

1. Mix the butter with paprika, seasoning and salt in a bowl.
2. Brush the chicken with this mixture and place it in a baking tray.
3. Cook in the preheated oven at 350F for 1¾ hours.
4. If needed, brush the chicken with the butter while cooking.
5. Serve the chicken warm.

Quick Zucchini Lasagna

Time: 1 hour
Servings: 6-8

Ingredients:

3 cups tomato sauce
1 teaspoon dried basil
½ teaspoon garlic powder
Salt and pepper to taste

4 zucchinis, sliced
2 cups shredded cooked chicken
1½ cups shredded mozzarella

Directions:

1. Mix the tomato sauce with basil and garlic powder, as well as salt and pepper in a bowl.
2. Layer the zucchini slices, tomato sauce and cooked chicken in a deep dish baking pan.
3. Top with mozzarella and cook in the preheated oven at 350F for 45-50 minutes.
4. Serve the lasagna warm.

Stuffed Bell Peppers

Time: 2 hours
Servings: 6

Ingredients:

2 tablespoons olive oil
2 sweet onions, chopped
1 carrot, grated
2 tablespoons tomato paste

1 pound ground pork
Salt and pepper to taste
6 red bell peppers, cored
4 cups vegetable stock

Directions:

1. Heat the oil in skillet and stir in the onions and carrot.
2. Sauté for 5 minutes then add the tomato paste and remove from heat.
3. Let the mixture cool slightly and stir in the pork.
4. Add salt and pepper to taste then stuff the bell peppers with this mixture.
5. Place the stuffed peppers in a deep saucepan and add the stock.
6. Cook on low heat for 1½ hours.
7. Serve the bell peppers warm.

Cajun Jumbo Prawns

Time: 30 minutes
Servings: 6

Ingredients:

18 jumbo prawns
2 tablespoons olive oil
2 tablespoons Cajun seasoning
½ cup grated Monterey Jack cheese

Directions:

1. Drizzle the prawns with olive oil and sprinkle with Cajun seasoning.
2. Heat a grill pan over medium to high flame and place the prawns on the grill.
3. Cook on both sides for 2-3 minutes then remove them from the grill and place them on a platter.
4. Top with a touch of cheese and serve the prawns warm.

Cauliflower Chicken Curry

Time: 1 hour
Servings: 4-6

Ingredients:

2 tablespoons vegetable oil
2 shallots, chopped
1 pound chicken breasts, cubed
2 tablespoons red curry paste
1 head cauliflower, cut into florets
1 cup chicken stock
2 cups water
½ cup coconut cream
½ lemongrass stalk, crushed
Salt and pepper to taste
Chopped cilantro for serving

Directions:

1. Heat the oil in a heavy pot and stir in the shallots.
2. Sauté for 2 minutes then add the chicken and cook 5 additional minutes.
3. Stir in the remaining ingredients and adjust the taste with salt and pepper.
4. Cook over low heat for 40 minutes and serve the curry warm, topped with chopped cilantro.

Pesto Chicken

Time: 1¼ hours
Servings: 4

Ingredients:

½ cup Italian pesto
4 chicken breasts
Salt and pepper to taste
½ cup chicken stock

Directions:

1. Spread the pesto over the chicken breasts and season with salt and pepper.
2. Place the chicken in a deep baking pan and add the stock.
3. Cook in the preheated oven at 350F for 30 minutes.
4. Serve the chicken warm.

Asian Slow Roasted Pork

Time: 6 hours
Servings: 6-8

Ingredients:

2 teaspoons grated ginger
¼ cup soy sauce
4 garlic cloves, minced
1 teaspoon onion powder
½ teaspoon dried oregano
½ teaspoon cayenne pepper
3 pounds pork shoulder

Directions:

1. Combine the ginger, soy sauce, garlic, onion powder, oregano and cayenne pepper in a bowl.
2. Spread this mixture over the piece of meat and rub it well into the meat.
3. Place the pork in a baking tray and top it with aluminum foil.
4. Cook in the preheated oven at 300F for 4 hours.
5. Remove the foil and cook on 350F for 1 additional hour.
6. Serve the pork warm with your favorite side dish.

Zucchini Pasta Bolognese

Time: 1 hour
Servings: 4-6

Ingredients:

2 tablespoons olive oil
1 pound ground beef
1 sweet onion, chopped
2 garlic cloves, minced
1 can diced tomatoes
Salt and pepper to taste
3 young zucchinis

Directions:

1. Heat the oil in a heavy saucepan and stir in the beef.
2. Sauté for 5 minutes then stir in the onion, garlic, tomatoes, salt and pepper.
3. Cook the sauce on low heat for 40 minutes.
4. To form the pasta, using a vegetable peeler, cut small ribbons of zucchini.
5. Place the zucchini pasta in a bowl and top with warm beef sauce.
6. Serve right away.

Lemon Zucchini Pasta

Time: 40 minutes
Servings: 4-6

Ingredients:

4 young zucchinis
1 cup cream cheese
1 tablespoon lemon zest
2 tablespoons lemon juice
¼ cup chopped parsley
2 tablespoons olive oil
¼ cup water
Salt and pepper to taste
2 cups cherry tomatoes, halved

Directions:

1. Using a vegetable peeler, cut thin ribbons of zucchini and place them in a salad bowl.
2. Combine the cream cheese, lemon zest, lemon juice, parsley, olive oil and water in a bowl.
3. Pour the cream cheese mixture over the zucchini and mix gently.
4. Season with salt and pepper to taste and top with cherry tomatoes before serving.

Shakshouka - Eggs in Tomato Sauce

Time: 40 minutes
Servings: 6

Ingredients:

- 2 tablespoons olive oil
- 1 shallot, chopped
- 1 garlic clove, chopped
- 1 teaspoon mustard seeds
- ½ teaspoon cumin seeds
- 1 can diced tomatoes
- 2 cups tomato sauce
- Salt and pepper to taste
- 6 eggs
- 2 tablespoons chopped parsley

Directions:

1. Heat the oil in a skillet and stir in the shallot and garlic.
2. Sauté for 2 minutes then stir in the mustard seeds, cumin seeds, tomatoes, tomato sauce, salt and pepper.
3. Cook the sauce on low heat for 10 minutes.
4. Crack open the eggs and drop them into the hot sauce.
5. Cover with a lid and cook on low heat for 10 additional minutes.
6. Serve the eggs topped with plenty of tomato sauce and garnished with parsley.

Lettuce Wrapped Scrambled Tofu

Time: 30 minutes
Servings: 4-6

Ingredients:

- 2 tablespoons vegetable oil
- 1 teaspoon turmeric powder
- ½ teaspoon cumin seeds
- ½ teaspoon fennel seeds
- ½ teaspoon mustard seeds
- 1 Thai red pepper, sliced
- 10 oz. firm tofu, crumbled
- 4-6 lettuce leaves

Directions:

1. Heat the oil in a skillet and stir in the turmeric, cumin, fennel seeds, mustard and Thai pepper.
2. Sauté for 1 minute then add the crumbled tofu and cook over medium flame for 10-15 minutes, stirring often.
3. Remove from heat and spoon the tofu into lettuce leaves.
4. Wrap tightly and serve fresh.

Roasted Turkey with Paprika Butter

Time: 1½ hours
Servings: 4-6

Ingredients:

¼ cup butter, softened
2 teaspoons smoked paprika
2 tablespoons tomato paste
2 garlic cloves, minced
Salt and pepper to taste
1½ pounds turkey breast
1 cup chicken stock

Directions:

1. Mix the butter, paprika, tomato paste and garlic in a bowl. Add salt and pepper to taste then spread this mixture over the turkey.
2. Place the turkey in a baking tray and add the stock into the tray as well.
3. Cook in the preheated oven at 350F for 1 hour.
4. It is ready when the juices run out clear.
5. Serve the turkey warm.

Asparagus Beef Stir-Fry

Time: 35 minutes
Servings: 2-4

Ingredients:

2 tablespoons vegetable oil
8 oz. beef steak, cut into thin strips
1 carrot, cut into sticks
8 asparagus strips, trimmed and coarsely sliced
¼ cup white wine
Salt and pepper to taste

Directions:

1. Heat the oil in a skillet or wok and stir in the beef strips.
2. Cook on medium to high flame for 10 minutes, stirring often.
3. Stir in the carrot and asparagus and cook 5 additional minutes.
4. Add the wine and cook until reduced then adjust the taste with salt and pepper.
5. Serve the stir-fry warm.

BBQ Ribs

Time: 2 hours
Servings: 4-6

Ingredients:

- 1½ cups BBQ sauce
- 1 teaspoon cumin powder
- 1 teaspoon garlic powder
- 1 teaspoon ground black pepper
- 1 teaspoon salt
- 3 pounds short ribs

Directions:

1. Combine the BBQ sauce with cumin, garlic powder, black pepper and salt in a bowl.
2. Add the short ribs and coat them evenly.
3. Place the ribs in a deep baking pan and cook in the preheated oven at 330F for 1½ hours.
4. Turn the heat on high and cook for 15 additional minutes.
5. Serve the ribs warm.

BBQ Pulled Pork

Time: 3¼ hours
Servings: 4-6

Ingredients:

- 2½ pounds pork shoulder
- 2 cups BBQ sauce
- 1 bay leaf
- 1 teaspoon salt
- 1 teaspoon cumin powder
- 1 teaspoon garlic powder
- ½ teaspoon onion powder

Directions:

1. Place the pork shoulder in a deep baking pan.
2. Mix the BBQ sauce with bay leaf, salt, cumin powder, garlic and onion powder in a bowl then spread the sauce over the pork.
3. Cook in the preheated oven at 300F for 2 hours then turn the heat on 375F and cook 1 additional hour.
4. When done, shred the pork into fine threads with two forks and serve in sandwiches.

Garlic Cheddar Chicken

Time: 1 hour
Servings: 4

Ingredients:

4 chicken breasts
1 cup almond meal
1 teaspoon garlic powder
1 teaspoon dried Italian herbs
1½ cups grated Cheddar

Directions:

1. Place the chicken breasts in a baking tray.
2. Mix the almond meal with garlic powder and herbs and spoon it over the chicken.
3. Top with grated cheese and cook in the preheated oven at 350F for 40-45 minutes or until golden brown and crusty.
4. Serve the chicken warm.

Paprika Parmesan Chicken

Time: 1 hour
Servings: 4

Ingredients:

½ cup grated Parmesan
½ cup almond meal
½ teaspoon salt
½ teaspoon smoked paprika
1 egg, beaten
2 tablespoons milk
4 chicken fillets
Oil for frying

Directions:

1. Mix the Parmesan with almond meal, salt and paprika in a bowl.
2. Mix the egg with milk.
3. Dip the chicken fillets into the egg then roll them through the almond mixture.
4. Heat the oil in a large skillet and place the chicken in the hot oil.
5. Fry on both sides for 6-8 minutes or until crisp and golden brown.
6. Serve the chicken fillets warm.

Baked Halibut Fillets with Zucchinis

Time: 45 minutes
Servings: 4

Ingredients:

½ shallot, chopped
1 teaspoon dried basil

1 teaspoon dried oregano
Salt and pepper to taste
4 halibut fillets

1 young zucchini, sliced
½ cup grated Parmesan

Directions:

1. Mix the shallot, basil, oregano, salt and pepper in a bowl.
2. Place the halibut fillets in a baking tray.
3. Top each fillet with a dollop of shallot mixture then arrange the zucchini slices on top.
4. Sprinkle with Parmesan and cook in the preheated oven at 350F for 25 minutes.
5. Serve the fish fillets warm.

Italian Style Fish Fillets

Time: 30 minutes
Servings: 4

Ingredients:

1½ pounds cod fillets, cubed
1 can diced tomatoes
1 shallot, chopped
1 garlic clove, minced

½ cup black olives, pitted
1 teaspoon Italian dried herbs
2 tablespoons olive oil
Salt and pepper to taste

Directions:

1. Combine all the ingredients in a deep dish baking pan.
2. Season with salt and pepper and cook in the preheated oven at 350F for 25 minutes.
3. Serve the fish warm.

Bacon Wrapped Pork Medallions

Time: 30 minutes
Servings: 4

Ingredients:

4 pork medallions
4 bacon slices
Salt and pepper to taste
2 tablespoons butter

2 tablespoons olive oil

Directions:

1. Wrap each pork medallion in bacon.
2. Season the medallions with salt and pepper.
3. Melt the butter and olive oil in a skillet.
4. Place the medallions in the hot oil and cook them on each side for 5-6 minutes.
5. When they are golden brown, fry the sides of the medallions as well until the bacon becomes slightly crisp.
6. Serve the pork medallions warm.

Burgundy Roasted Pork

Time: 1¾ hours
Servings: 4-6

Ingredients:

1 celery stalk, sliced
1 red onion, sliced
1½ cups burgundy wine
2 pounds pork shoulder
1 teaspoon onion powder
1 teaspoon garlic powder
1 teaspoon dried thyme
1 teaspoon salt

Directions:

1. Mix the celery, red onion and wine in a deep dish baking pan.
2. Sprinkle the pork with onion, garlic powder, thyme and salt then place it in the pan.
3. Cook in the preheated oven at 350F for 1½ hours.
4. Serve the pork warm with your favorite side dish.

Garlicky Roasted Pork Loin

Time: 1¾ hours
Servings: 4-6

Ingredients:

6 garlic cloves, minced
1 teaspoon smoked paprika
1 teaspoon sweet paprika
2 tablespoons olive oil
1 teaspoon salt
2 pounds boneless pork loin

Directions:

1. Mix the garlic, paprika, olive oil and salt in a bowl.

2. Spread this mixture over the pork loin and rub it well into the meat.
3. Place the meat in a baking tray and cover it with aluminum foil.
4. Cook in the preheated oven at 350F for 1 hour then remove the foil and cook 30 additional minutes.
5. Serve the pork warm.

BBQ Cumin Roasted Ribs

Time: 2 hours
Servings: 4-6

Ingredients:

2 teaspoons cumin powder
1 cup BBQ sauce
1 teaspoon chili powder
1 teaspoon smoked paprika
1 teaspoon salt
3 pounds baby back ribs

Directions:

1. Mix the cumin powder, BBQ sauce, chili powder, paprika and salt in a bowl.
2. Add the baby back ribs and toss them around to evenly coat them.
3. Place the ribs in a baking pan and pour the sauce over them.
4. Cook in the preheated oven at 330F for 1½ hours.
5. Cook 15 additional minutes on highest heat and serve the ribs warm.

Blue Cheese Pork Chops

Time: 40 minutes
Servings: 4

Ingredients:

4 pork chops
Salt and pepper to taste
2 tablespoons butter
2 tablespoons vegetable oil
¼ cup crumbled blue cheese
¼ cup cream cheese

Directions:

1. Season the pork chops with salt and pepper.
2. Heat the butter and oil in a skillet then place the pork chops in the hot oil.
3. Cook on each side for 5-7 minutes or until golden brown.
4. To serve, mix the blue cheese with cream cheese.

5. Place the pork chops on serving plates and top with a dollop of blue cheese mixture.
6. Serve immediately.

Onion Salmon Patties

Time: 35 minutes
Servings: 4-6

Ingredients:

3 salmon fillets
1 egg
2 green onions, chopped
1 tablespoon chopped dill
Salt and pepper to taste
½ cup almond meal
¼ cup vegetable oil for frying

Directions:

1. Place the salmon in a food processor and pulse until ground.
2. Stir in the egg, green onions, dill, salt and pepper and mix well.
3. Heat the oil in a deep frying pan.
4. Form small patties and roll them through almond meal.
5. Place the patties in the hot oil and fry on both sides for 2-3 minutes or until golden brown.
6. Remove them on paper towels and serve them warm.

Lemon Pork Loin Cooked in Oil Bath

Time: 2 hours
Servings: 2-4

Ingredients:

1½ pounds pork loin
Salt and pepper to taste
2 cups vegetable oil
1 lemon, juiced

Directions:

1. Season the pork loin with salt and pepper and place it in a deep heavy saucepan.
2. Add the oil and lemon juice then cover the saucepan with aluminum foil, topped with a lid to seal it well.
3. Cook over low heat for 1½ hours.
4. Serve the pork loin warm with your favorite side dish.

Lemon Pepper Pork Chops

Time: 1 hour
Servings: 4

Ingredients:

¼ cup butter, softened
4 pork chops
Salt and pepper to taste
4 slices lemon
2 jalapeño peppers, chopped

Directions:

1. Spread the butter over each pork chop.
2. Season with salt and pepper then take 4 sheets of aluminum foil.
3. Place each pork chop in the center of the aluminum sheets and top each chop with a slice of lemon and a few bits of jalapeño.
4. Wrap the pork chops well and place them in a baking tray.
5. Cook in the preheated oven at 350F for 30 minutes.
6. Serve the pork chops warm.

Ginger Pork Stir-Fry

Time: 35 minutes
Servings: 2-4

Ingredients:

2 tablespoons vegetable oil
1 teaspoon grated ginger
1 teaspoon minced garlic
½ pound pork loin, cut into thin strips
4 Portobello mushrooms, sliced
1 tablespoon dark soy sauce
1 green onion, chopped
Salt and pepper to taste

Directions:

1. Heat the vegetable oil in a wok and stir in the ginger and garlic.
2. Sauté for 30 seconds then add the pork loin.
3. Cook for 5 minutes on high heat then stir in the mushrooms.
4. Cook 10 additional minutes, stirring often then add the soy sauce and green onion and keep over flame for a few more minutes. Add salt and pepper to taste.
5. Serve the stir-fry warm.

Bacon Wrapped Pork Loin

Time: 2½ hours
Servings: 8-10

Ingredients:

4 garlic cloves, minced
1 teaspoon dried basil
1 teaspoon smoked paprika
½ teaspoon salt

4 pounds pork loin roast
1 cup vegetable stock
1 bay leaf
12 slices bacon

Directions:

1. Mix the garlic, basil, paprika and salt in a bowl then spread this mixture over the pork and rub it well into the meat.
2. Place the pork in a deep dish baking pan.
3. Add the stock and bay leaf into the pan then top the pork with slices of bacon.
4. Cook in the preheated oven at 330F for 1½ hours and on 375F for 30 minutes.
5. Serve the pork loin warm with your favorite side dish.

Sausage and Zucchini Stew

Time: 40 minutes
Servings: 4-6

Ingredients:

1 tablespoon olive oil
4 smoked sausages, sliced
1 sweet onion, sliced
1 garlic clove, minced
4 young zucchinis, sliced

1 can diced tomatoes
1 bay leaf
½ teaspoon dried oregano
Salt and pepper to taste

Directions:

1. Heat the oil in a heavy saucepan and stir in the sausages.
2. Cook for 5 minutes then stir in the onion and garlic and sauté for 2 minutes.
3. Add the zucchinis, tomatoes, bay leaf and oregano, as well as salt and pepper to taste.
4. Cook the stew over low heat for 30 minutes.
5. Serve the stew warm.

Sauerkraut Pork Chops

Time: 1 hour
Servings: 4

Ingredients:

1 pound sauerkraut, shredded
1 red onion, sliced
1 bay leaf
2 ripe tomatoes, sliced
1 teaspoon dried thyme
4 pork chops
Salt and pepper to taste

Directions:

1. Mix the sauerkraut with onion, bay leaf, tomatoes and thyme in a deep dish baking pan.
2. Season the pork chops with salt and pepper and place them over the sauerkraut.
3. Cook in the preheated oven at 330F for 40 minutes.
4. Serve them warm.

Ham Cooked in Beer

Time: 6 hours
Servings: 8-10

Ingredients:

5-pound piece of ham
3 bay leaves
4 cups beer

Directions:

1. Place the ham in a deep dish baking pan.
2. Add the beer and bay leaves and cover with aluminum foil.
3. Cook in the preheated oven at 300F for 4 hours then remove the foil and cook on 350F for 2 additional hours.
4. Serve the ham warm with your favorite side dish.

Bacon Wrapped Pesto Chicken

Time: 1 hour
Servings: 4

Ingredients:

¼ cup pesto
4 chicken breasts
¼ cup grated Parmesan
8 bacon slices

Directions:

1. Spread the pesto over each chicken breast and sprinkle them with grated cheese.
2. Wrap each chicken breast into 2 slices of bacon and place them in a small baking tray.
3. Cook in the preheated oven at 350F for 30 minutes.
4. Serve the chicken warm.

Grilled Salmon with Wasabi Sauce

Time: 35 minutes
Servings: 4

Ingredients:

4 salmon fillets
Salt and pepper to taste
2 tablespoons butter
1 small shallot, finely chopped
¼ cup dry white wine
1 cup chopped cilantro
1 tablespoon wasabi paste
½ cup heavy cream

Directions:

1. Season the salmon with salt and pepper and cook it over a heated grill pan for 4-5 minutes on each side.
2. To make the sauce, melt the butter in a small saucepan.
3. Add the shallot and sauté for 5 minutes on low heat.
4. Stir in the wine, cilantro and wasabi paste and cook the sauce for 5 additional minutes.
5. Stir in the heavy cream and remove from heat.
6. Serve the grilled salmon topped with wasabi sauce.

Marinated Grilled Tuna

Time: 40 minutes
Servings: 4

Ingredients:

4 garlic cloves, sliced
¼ cup white wine

2 tablespoons lemon juice
½ teaspoon wasabi paste
1 tablespoon soy sauce

2 tablespoons chopped cilantro
½ teaspoon salt
4 tuna steaks

Directions:

1. Mix the garlic, wine, lemon juice, wasabi paste, soy sauce, cilantro and salt in a bowl.
2. Add the tuna steaks and toss them around to coat them in marinade.
3. Marinate the steaks for 20 minutes.
4. Heat a grill pan over medium to high flame then place the tuna steaks on the grill.
5. Cook on each side for 3-4 minutes just until you can see the grill marks.
6. Serve the tuna steaks warm with your favorite side dish.

Three Meat Meatballs

Time: 1 hour
Servings: 6-8

Ingredients:

1 pound ground beef
1 pound ground pork
1 pound ground chicken
1 carrot, grated
3 garlic cloves, minced

2 tablespoons chopped cilantro
2 eggs
¼ cup almond meal
Salt and pepper to taste

Directions:

1. Combine all the ingredients in a bowl.
2. Add salt and pepper to taste and mix well.
3. Wet your hands and form small meatballs.
4. Place them on a baking tray lined with parchment paper and cook in the preheated oven at 350F for 25 minutes or until golden brown.
5. Let them cool in the pan before serving.

Grilled Pork Chops with Asian Style Sauce

Time: 45 minutes
Servings: 4

Ingredients:

2 green onions, chopped
½ teaspoon grated ginger
¼ cup soy sauce
1 teaspoon honey

1 pinch chili powder
4 pork chops
Salt and pepper to taste

Directions:

1. Mix the green onions, ginger, soy sauce, honey and chili powder in a bowl.
2. Season the pork chops with salt and pepper.
3. Heat a grill pan over medium flame.
4. Place the pork chops on the grill and cook them on each side for 4-5 minutes.
5. Serve the grilled pork chops drizzled with the sauce you made earlier.

Allspice Spare Ribs

Time: 2¼ hours
Servings: 6

Ingredients:

1½ cups beef stock
1 tablespoon maple syrup
2 teaspoons salt

¼ cup melted butter
2 teaspoons allspice powder
3 pounds pork ribs

Directions:

1. Mix the stock with the maple syrup, salt, butter and allspice and pour it into a deep dish baking pan.
2. Add the spare ribs and cook them in the preheated oven at 350F for 2 hours.
3. Serve the spare ribs warm.

Pork Chops with Sautéed Fennel

Time: 45 minutes
Servings: 4

Ingredients:

4 pork chops
Salt and pepper to taste
1 fennel bulb, sliced
2 tablespoons butter

1 tablespoon olive oil
1 garlic clove, minced
1 tablespoon balsamic vinegar

Directions:

1. Season the pork chops with salt and pepper.
2. Heat a grill pan over medium flame and place the pork chops on the grill.
3. Cook the pork chops on each side for 5-6 minutes.
4. To make the sautéed fennel, melt the butter in a skillet.
5. Add the oil and garlic then stir in the fennel.
6. Cook for 10 minutes, stirring often, until softened.
7. Add the balsamic vinegar and remove from heat.
8. Serve the pork chops topped with sautéed fennel.

Carne con Chilies

Time: 2¼ hours
Servings: 8-10

Ingredients:

3 tablespoons vegetable oil
2 pounds ground pork
2 onions, chopped
4 garlic cloves, minced
4 jalapeño peppers, chopped

4 tomatillos, chopped
1 can diced tomatoes
1 red dried chili, chopped
Salt and pepper to taste

Directions:

1. Heat the oil in a heavy saucepan and stir in the ground pork.
2. Cook for 10 minutes, stirring often, then add the onions, garlic, jalapeños, tomatillos, tomatoes and chili.
3. Season with salt and pepper and cook on low heat for 2 hours.
4. Serve the carne con chilies warm, preferably with pita bread.

Cajun Catfish

Time: 1½ hours
Servings: 4-6

Ingredients:

1½ pounds catfish fillets, cut into strips
Salt and pepper to taste
2 tablespoons Cajun seasoning

4 tablespoons butter
½ cup chopped parsley
2 green onions, chopped

1 can condensed cream of mushroom soup

Directions:

1. Season the fish strips with salt, pepper and Cajun seasoning.
2. Melt of the butter in a skillet and stir in the parsley, green onions and mushroom soup.
3. Cook for 10 minutes then stir in the fish strips.
4. Cook on low heat for 20 minutes.
5. Remove from heat and serve the fish warm.

Poached Salmon with Piccata Sauce

Time: 40 minutes
Servings: 4

Ingredients:

4 cups water
4 lemon slices
Salt and pepper to taste
4 salmon fillets

¼ cup mayonnaise
1 teaspoon capers, chopped
2 tablespoons chopped parsley

Directions:

1. Combine the water with lemon, salt and pepper in a saucepan and bring to a boil.
2. Place the salmon fillets in the boiling water and cook for 15 minutes.
3. For the sauce, mix the mayonnaise with capers and parsley.
4. Drizzle the warm poached salmon fillets with piccata sauce and serve them warm.

Spicy Fried Cod

Time: 30 minutes
Servings: 4

Ingredients:

2 tablespoons all-purpose flour
1½ teaspoons hot paprika
1 teaspoon salt
4 cod fillets
1 cup vegetable oil for frying

Directions:

1. Mix the flour with hot paprika and salt in a bowl.
2. Sprinkle the cod fillets with the flour mixture.
3. Hot the oil in a deep frying pan then place the cod fillets into the hot oil.
4. Fry on both sides until golden brown and serve the cod fillets warm.

Roasted Trout with Yogurt Sauce

Time: 45 minutes
Servings: 2

Ingredients:

2 whole trouts, cleaned
2 lemon sliced
¼ bunch parsley
Salt and pepper to taste

½ cup plain yogurt
2 garlic cloves, minced
2 tablespoons chopped parsley

Directions:

1. Stuff the trouts with lemon slices and parsley then season them with salt and pepper.
2. Place the trouts in a baking tray and cook in the preheated oven at 350F for 30 minutes.
3. For the sauce, mix the yogurt, garlic and parsley in a bowl. Adjust the taste with salt and pepper.
4. Serve the trouts drizzled with the yogurt sauce.

BBQ Slow Cooker Brisket

Time: 10¼ hours
Servings: 10

Ingredients:

1½ cups BBQ sauce
1 teaspoon garlic powder
½ teaspoon celery seeds
2 tablespoons Worcestershire sauce
1 teaspoon mustard seeds
1 teaspoon salt
¼ cup water

4 pounds beef brisket

Directions:

1. Mix the BBQ sauce with garlic, celery seeds, Worcestershire sauce, mustard seeds, salt and water in a bowl.
2. Place the brisket in a slow cooker then cover it with the sauce.
3. Cook on low settings for 10 hours.
4. Serve the brisket warm.

Grilled Salmon with Lemon and Tarragon Sauce

Time: 35 minutes
Servings: 4

Ingredients:

4 salmon fillets
Salt and pepper to taste
½ cup mayonnaise
2 teaspoons dried tarragon
3 tablespoons lemon juice
1 tablespoon Dijon mustard

Directions:

1. Season the salmon fillets with salt and pepper to taste.
2. Heat a grill pan over medium flame and place the salmon on the hot grill.
3. Cook the salmon on each side for 4-5 minutes until browned.
4. For the sauce, combine the mayonnaise with tarragon, lemon juice and mustard. Add salt and pepper to taste.
5. Serve the salmon fillets drizzled with the tarragon sauce.

Blue Cheese Stuffed Pork Chops

Time: 45 minutes
Servings: 4

Ingredients:

4 pork chops
½ cup crumbled blue cheese
½ teaspoon dried thyme
Salt and pepper to taste

Directions:

1. Cut a small hole into each pork chop.
2. Mix the blue cheese with thyme then stuff each pork chop with the blue cheese mixture.

3. Season the pork chops with salt and pepper and cook in the preheated oven for 30 minutes.
4. Serve the pork chops warm.

Pepperoncini Beef

Time: 6¼ hours
Servings: 8-10

Ingredients:

1 jar pepperoncini, chopped
4 garlic cloves, chopped
Salt and pepper to taste
3 pounds beef chuck roast, cut into large cubes
1 cup grated Provolone cheese

Directions:

1. Mix the pepperoncini with garlic, salt and pepper in a deep dish baking pan.
2. Stir in the chuck roast.
3. Cover with grated cheese and cook in the preheated oven at 300F for 6 hours.
4. Serve the beef warm.

Cheeseburger Meatloaf

Time: 1¼ hours
Servings: 8-10

Ingredients:

2 pounds ground beef
1 shallot, chopped
Salt and pepper to taste
2 eggs
¼ cup chopped fresh herbs of your choice
½ teaspoon cumin powder
½ teaspoon chili powder
2 cups grated Cheddar

Directions:

1. Mix the ground beef with shallot, salt, pepper, eggs, herbs, cumin powder and chili powder in a bowl.
2. Spoon half if the meat mixture into a loaf pan lined with parchment paper.
3. Top with half of the cheese and spoon the remaining meat over the cheese.
4. Cover with the other half of cheese and cook in the preheated oven at 350F for 40-45 minutes.
5. Serve the meatloaf warm.

Beef Steak with Garlic Wine Sauce

Time: 1¼ hours
Servings: 4

Ingredients:

4 beef steak
Salt and pepper to taste
4 tablespoons butter
1 garlic clove, crushed
1 cup dry red wine

Directions:

1. Season the steaks with salt and pepper to taste.
2. Melt the butter in a skillet and add the garlic. Sauté for 30 seconds then remove and discard the garlic.
3. Place the beef steaks into the hot oil and fry them on each side for 4-5 minutes.
4. Pour in the wine and cook on high heat for 10-15 minutes.
5. Serve the steaks warm, drizzled with wine sauce.

Coffee Roasted Beef

Time: 3¼ hours
Servings: 6-8

Ingredients:

4 garlic cloves, minced
1 cup strong coffee
1 teaspoon salt
1 teaspoon chili powder
3 pounds beef chuck roast

Directions:

1. Mix the garlic with coffee, salt and chili powder.
2. Place the beef in a deep baking pan then pour in the coffee mixture.
3. Cook in the preheated oven at 300F for 2 hours then on 350F for 1 additional hour.
4. Serve the beef warm.

Szechuan Beef

Time: 3¼ hours
Servings: 6-8

Ingredients:

- 1 can water chestnuts, drained
- ¼ cup soy sauce
- 3 garlic cloves, minced
- 2 teaspoons Szechuan pepper
- 2 green onions, finely chopped
- 2½ pounds beef roast
- Salt and pepper to taste

Directions:

1. Place the water chestnuts in a deep baking pan.
2. Mix the soy sauce, garlic, Szechuan pepper and green onions in a bowl.
3. Spread this mixture over the beef and rub it well into the meat. Add salt and pepper to taste.
4. Place the meat over the chestnuts and cook in the preheated oven at 300F for 1½ hours then turn the heat on 350F and cook 1 additional hour.
5. Serve the beef and chestnuts warm.

Sloppy Joe Casserole

Time: 1¼ hours
Servings: 6-8

Ingredients:

- 2 tablespoons vegetable oil
- 2 sweet onions, sliced
- 2 pounds ground beef
- 1 celery stalk, sliced
- 2 garlic cloves, minced
- ½ cup tomato sauce
- 1 cup diced tomatoes
- 1 tablespoon apple cider vinegar
- 1 tablespoon Splenda
- 1 teaspoon Dijon mustard
- Salt and pepper to taste
- 2 cups grated Cheddar

Directions:

1. Heat the oil in a skillet and stir in the onions.
2. Sauté for 5 minutes then stir in the beef and cook 5 additional minutes.
3. Stir in the celery, garlic, tomato sauce, diced tomatoes, vinegar, Splenda and mustard.
4. Season with salt and pepper to taste.
5. Pour the mixture into a deep dish baking pan and top with grated cheese.
6. Cook in the preheated oven at 350F for 40 minutes.
7. Serve the casserole warm.

Spicy Marinated Beef Steaks

Time: 1½ hours
Servings: 4

Ingredients:

4 beef steaks
¼ cup soy sauce
2 tablespoons olive oil
2 red peppers, chopped
1 teaspoon grated ginger
1 green onion, chopped
½ teaspoon sesame oil

Directions:

1. Combine all the ingredients in a zip-lock bag.
2. Seal the bag and let them marinate for 1 hour.
3. Heat a grill pan over medium flame then place the beef steaks on the grill.
4. Cook them on each side for 5-7 minutes until browned.
5. Serve the steaks warm.

Tomato Cabbage Stew

Time: 1 hour
Servings: 4-6

Ingredients:

2 tablespoons olive oil
1 head cabbage, shredded
1 red onion, chopped
1 carrot, grated
1 can diced tomatoes
Salt and pepper to taste
½ teaspoon dried thyme

Directions:

1. Heat the olive oil in a heavy pot.
2. Add the cabbage, onion, carrot, tomatoes, salt and pepper and cook on medium flame for 40 minutes.
3. Serve the stew warm, topped with thyme.

Cheesy Ham Quiche

Time: 1 hour
Servings: 6-8

Ingredients:

1 cup diced ham
4 eggs, beaten
1 cup heavy cream
1 cup grated Cheddar
1 tablespoon chopped chives
Salt and pepper to taste
Butter to grease the pan

Directions:

1. Combine all the ingredients in a bowl.
2. Grease the pan with butter and pour the quiche mixture into the pan.
3. Cook in the preheated oven at 350F for 35 minutes.
4. Serve the quiche warm.

Sherry Braised Beef

Time: 2½ hours
Servings: 6-8

Ingredients:

2 garlic cloves, chopped
1 cup dry sherry
1 bay leaf
½ cup beef stock
Salt and pepper to taste
3 pounds beef roast

Directions:

1. Mix the garlic, sherry, bay leaf, stock, salt and pepper in a deep dish baking pan.
2. Add the beef roast in the pan as well and cook in the preheated oven at 350F for 2 hours, pouring some of the sauce in the pan over the beef from time to time.
3. Serve the beef warm.

Cheesy Pork and Cauliflower Casserole

Time: 1¼ hours
Servings: 6-8

Ingredients:

1½ pounds pork, cubed
1 head cauliflower, cut into florets
1 cup cream cheese
1 cup vegetable stock
Salt and pepper to taste
1 cup grated Cheddar

Directions:

1. Mix the pork and cauliflower in a deep dish baking pan.
2. Combine the cream cheese and stock in a bowl and pour the mixture over the pork and cauliflower.
3. Sprinkle with salt and pepper and top with cheese.
4. Cook in the preheated oven at 350F for 45 minutes.
5. Serve the casserole warm.

Side Dishes

Cauliflower Rice

Time: 50 minutes
Servings: 4-6

Ingredients:

2 tablespoons butter
1 carrot, diced
1 shallot, chopped
1 red bell pepper, cored and diced
1 yellow bell pepper, cored and diced
1 head cauliflower
1 cup vegetable stock
Salt and pepper to taste
2 tablespoons chopped cilantro

Directions:

1. Melt the butter in a skillet and stir in the carrot, shallot and bell peppers.
2. Sauté for 5 minutes.
3. Place the cauliflower in a food processor and pulse until ground, but not too fine.
4. Spoon the cauliflower rice into the skillet and stir in the stock. Add salt and pepper to taste and cook the cauliflower rice for 15-20 minutes.
5. Serve the rice warm, topped with chopped cilantro.

Festive Sautéed Onions

Time: 45 minutes
Servings: 4-6

Ingredients:

2 tablespoons butter
1 tablespoon olive oil
6 red onions, sliced
1 cup heavy cream
Salt and pepper to taste
½ cup grated Parmesan

Directions:

1. Heat the butter and oil in a skillet and stir in the red onions.
2. Sauté for 15 minutes, stirring often.
3. Remove from heat and transfer the mixture in a deep dish baking pan.
4. Stir in the cream, salt and pepper and top with grated cheese.
5. Cook in the preheated oven at 375F for 15 minutes.
6. Serve the onions warm.

Creamy Spinach

Time: 30 minutes
Servings: 2-4

Ingredients:

2 tablespoons olive oil
1 garlic clove, minced
1 shallot, chopped
1 pound fresh spinach, shredded
1 cup cream cheese
½ cup vegetable stock
Salt and pepper to taste

Directions:

1. Heat the oil in a skillet and stir in the garlic and shallot and sauté for 2 minutes.
2. Stir in the spinach and cook for 10 minutes, stirring often.
3. Add the cream cheese, stock, salt and pepper and cook 10 additional minutes.
4. Serve the spinach warm.

Roasted Cauliflower with Tomato Sauce

Time: 1¼ hours
Servings: 4-6

Ingredients:

2 cups tomato sauce
½ cup chicken stock
1 teaspoon dried basil
½ teaspoon dried oregano
1 teaspoon salt
½ teaspoon cumin powder
¼ teaspoon chili flakes
1 head cauliflower

Directions:

1. Mix the tomato sauce, chicken stock, basil, oregano, salt, cumin powder and chili flakes in a bowl.
2. Place the whole cauliflower head in a deep heavy pot that can go in the oven.
3. Pour the tomato sauce mixture over the cauliflower and cover the pot with a lid.
4. Cook in the preheated oven at 350F for 45 minutes.
5. Serve the cauliflower warm.

Almond Butter Broccoli Bake

Time: 40 minutes

Servings: 2-4

Ingredients:

½ cup almond butter, softened
2 tablespoons lemon juice
Salt and pepper to taste
2 pounds broccoli, cut into florets
¼ cup sliced almonds

Directions:

1. Mix the almond butter with lemon juice, salt and pepper in a bowl.
2. Place the broccoli in a baking tray then drizzle the florets with almond butter and toss them around to evenly coat them.
3. Sprinkle with sliced almonds and cook in the preheated oven at 350F for 20-25 minutes.
4. Serve the broccoli warm.

Balsamic Grilled Zucchini

Time: 45 minutes
Servings: 2-4

Ingredients:

3 tablespoons butter, melted
2 garlic cloves, minced
Salt and pepper to taste
2 zucchinis, sliced
3 tablespoons balsamic vinegar

Directions:

1. Mix the melted butter with garlic, salt and pepper and brush the zucchini slices with this mixture.
2. Heat a grill pan over medium flame and place the zucchini slices on the grill.
3. Cook on both sides until golden brown then transfer the zucchinis in a bowl and drizzle with balsamic vinegar.
4. Serve the zucchinis warm or chilled.

Lemon Sautéed Zucchini

Time: 35 minutes
Servings: 2-4

Ingredients:

3 tablespoons olive oil
1 tablespoon butter
2 garlic cloves, minced
3 young zucchinis, sliced
½ lemon, juiced
¼ cup chopped cilantro
Salt and pepper to taste

Directions:

1. Heat the oil and butter in a skillet and stir in the garlic.
2. Sauté for 30 seconds then add the zucchinis.
3. Cook for 10 minutes then stir in the lemon juice and cilantro, as well as salt and pepper to taste.
4. Keep cooking for 10 additional minutes and serve the dish warm.

Crispy Cabbage

Time: 45 minutes
Servings: 4-6

Ingredients:

4 tablespoons butter
1 tablespoon olive oil
1 head cabbage, shredded
Salt and pepper to taste

Directions:

1. Melt the butter and oil in a large skillet and stir in the cabbage.
2. Cook for 20 minutes, stirring all the time.
3. Season with salt and pepper and serve the cabbage warm.

Lemony Green Beans

Time: 50 minutes
Servings: 4-6

Ingredients:

2 pounds green beans, trimmed
3 tablespoons olive oil
2 garlic cloves, crushed
½ lemon, juiced
Salt and pepper to taste

Directions:

1. Pour a few cups of water in a large pot and bring it to a boil with a pinch of salt.
2. When the water is boiling, throw in the beans and blanch them for 15 minutes.
3. Drain and place aside.
4. Heat the oil in a large skillet and add the garlic. Sauté for 1 minute then remove the garlic.
5. Add the beans into the skillet and cook, stirring often for 10 minutes.
6. Drizzle with lemon juice and adjust the taste with salt and pepper.
7. Serve the beans warm.

Garlicky Spinach

Time: 35 minutes
Servings: 2-4

Ingredients:

4 tablespoons olive oil
3 garlic cloves, sliced
1½ pounds fresh spinach, trimmed and shredded
Salt and pepper to taste

Directions:

1. Heat the oil in a large skillet.
2. Add the garlic and sauté for 30 seconds then stir in the spinach.
3. Cook for 10-15 minutes until softened.
4. Add salt and pepper to taste. Serve the spinach warm.

Lime Drizzled Spinach

Time: 35 minutes
Servings: 2-4

Ingredients:

1 tablespoon butter
2 tablespoons olive oil
2 garlic cloves, chopped
1½ pounds fresh spinach, trimmed and shredded
Salt and pepper to taste
1 lime, juiced
Parmesan shavings for serving

Directions:

1. Heat the butter and oil in a large skillet.
2. Stir in the garlic and sauté for 30 seconds.
3. Stir in the spinach and cook for 10-15 minutes, until softened.
4. When done, adjust the taste with salt and pepper and drizzle with lime juice.
5. Serve topped with Parmesan shavings.

Balsamic Spinach and Onion Sauté

Time: 45 minutes
Servings: 2-4

Ingredients:

2 tablespoons butter
2 tablespoons olive oil
4 red onions, sliced
1 pound fresh spinach
Salt and pepper to taste
2 tablespoons balsamic vinegar

Directions:

1. Heat the butter and oil in a skillet and stir in the onions.
2. Cook the onions for 10 minutes until softened and slightly browned.
3. Stir in the spinach and cook 10 additional minutes then adjust the taste with salt and pepper and drizzle with balsamic vinegar.
4. Serve the dish warm.

Italian Style Spinach

Time: 45 minutes
Servings: 2-4

Ingredients:

2 tablespoons olive oil
1 pound fresh spinach, shredded
6 fresh figs, quartered
1 teaspoon dried Italian herbs
Salt and pepper to taste
2 tablespoons balsamic vinegar

Directions:

1. Heat the oil in a skillet.
2. Stir in the spinach and sauté for 10 minutes.

3. Stir in the figs and herbs then add salt and pepper to taste and cook 10 additional minutes on low heat.
4. Drizzle with balsamic vinegar before serving.

Garlic Mashed Potatoes

Time: 1½ hours
Servings: 4-6

Ingredients:

2 garlic heads
2 pounds potatoes, peeled and cubed
Pinch of salt
2 tablespoons butter
2 tablespoons heavy cream
¼ cup whole milk
¼ cup grated Parmesan
Salt and pepper to taste

Directions:

1. Cut the garlic heads in half lengthwise and wrap each half in aluminum foil.
2. Place the wrapped garlic in a baking tray and cook in the preheated oven at 350F for 40 minutes.
3. While the garlic cooks, place the potatoes in a pot and cover them with water.
4. Add a pinch of salt and cook the potatoes until tender.
5. Remove the garlic from the oven and carefully squeeze the cooked garlic into a bowl (make sure no skin is left into the bowl).
6. Drain the potatoes and place them in the bowl as well.
7. Mash the potatoes and garlic with a potato masher.
8. Stir in the butter, cream and milk, then add the cheese.
9. Adjust the taste with salt and pepper and serve the mashed potatoes warm.

Cheesy Broccoli Casserole

Time: 1¼ hours
Servings: 4-6

Ingredients:

4 bacon slices, chopped
1 sweet onion, sliced
2 garlic cloves, minced
1½ pounds broccoli, cut into florets
½ cup water
1½ cups grated Cheddar

Directions:

1. Heat a skillet over medium flame and stir in the bacon. Cook until crisp then stir in the onion and garlic.
2. Sauté for 2 additional minutes then stir in the broccoli.
3. Cook 5 more minutes then transfer the broccoli in a deep dish baking pan.
4. Add the water and top with cheese.
5. Cook in the preheated oven at 350F for 30-40 minutes or until golden brown and crusty on top.
6. Serve the casserole warm.

Parmesan Zucchini Sticks

Time: 45 minutes
Servings: 2-4

Ingredients:

½ cup almond meal
½ cup grated Parmesan
½ teaspoon dried basil
2 large zucchinis, cut into sticks
½ cup plain yogurt

Directions:

1. Mix the almond meal, Parmesan and basil in a bowl.
2. Dip the zucchinis into yogurt first then roll them through the almond and Parmesan mixture.
3. Place all the sticks in a baking tray lined with parchment paper and bake in the preheated oven at 350F for 20 minutes or until golden brown.
4. Serve them warm or chilled.

Fried Zucchini Slices

Time: 45 minutes
Servings: 4-6

Ingredients:

1 cup almond flour
1 teaspoon salt
½ teaspoon ground black pepper
Oil for frying
2 large zucchinis, sliced
2 eggs, beaten

Directions:

1. Mix the flour, salt and black pepper in a bowl.
2. Heat enough oil in a deep frying pan.
3. Dip the zucchini slices in beaten egg then roll them through the flour mixture.
4. Drop the zucchini slices in the hot oil and fry them on both sides until golden brown.
5. Remove them on paper towels.
6. Serve the zucchini slices warm.

Sautéed Broccoli Rabe

Time: 40 minutes
Servings: 4-6

Ingredients:

3 tablespoons olive oil
1 tablespoon butter
1 garlic clove, crushed
2 pounds broccoli rabe
½ cup grated Parmesan

Directions:

1. Heat the oil and butter in a skillet.
2. Add the garlic and sauté for 30 seconds then remove and discard the garlic.
3. Stir in the broccoli rabe and cook for 15-20 minutes, stirring often.
4. Remove from heat and sprinkle with Parmesan before serving.

Buttered Mushrooms

Time: 30 minutes
Servings: 2-4

Ingredients:

4 tablespoons butter
1 garlic clove, crushed
6 Portobello mushrooms, sliced
Salt and pepper to taste
1 tablespoon chopped cilantro

Directions:

1. Melt the butter in a skillet and stir in the garlic.
2. Sauté for 1 minute until golden brown then remove the garlic.

3. Add the mushroom slices, as well as salt and pepper and cook for 15-20 minutes, stirring often, until most of the liquid has evaporated.
4. Serve the mushrooms warm, topped with chopped cilantro.

Desserts

Peach Cobbler

Time: 45 minutes
Servings: 4-6

Ingredients:

6 ripe peaches, pitted and sliced
1 teaspoon cinnamon powder
¼ cup chilled butter, cubed
1 cup almond flour
1 pinch salt
¼ cup Splenda
¼ cup cold buttermilk

Directions:

1. Mix the peaches with cinnamon in a deep dish baking pan.
2. Combine the butter, almond flour, salt and Splenda in bowl and rub them well together.
3. Stir in the buttermilk then spoon the batter over the peaches.
4. Cook in the preheated oven at 350F for 30 minutes.
5. Serve the cobbler chilled.

Coconut Almond Bread

Time: 1 hour
Servings: 6-8

Ingredients:

8 eggs
½ cup Splenda powder
1½ cups almond flour
¼ cup coconut flour
¼ cup ground flax seeds
½ cup coconut flakes
1 teaspoon baking soda
1 pinch salt

Directions:

1. Whip the eggs with the Splenda until stiff.
2. Stir in the dry ingredients then pour the batter into a loaf pan lined with parchment paper.
3. Bake in the preheated oven at 350F for 40 minutes or until golden brown and well risen.
4. Let the bread cool in the pan before serving.

Chocolate Walnut Candy

Time: 35 minutes
Servings: 4-6

Ingredients:

8 oz. dark chocolate, chopped
2 teaspoons coconut oil
1½ cups walnuts, roasted and coarsely chopped
¼ teaspoon sea salt

Directions:

1. Melt the chocolate and coconut oil in a heatproof bowl over a hot water bath until smooth.
2. Remove from heat and spread the mixture over a baking sheet.
3. Top with walnuts and a sprinkle of sea salt and refrigerate for 20 minutes until set.
4. Break into smaller pieces and serve fresh.

Orange Chocolate Truffles

Time: 45 minutes
Servings: 6-8

Ingredients:

⅔ cup heavy cream
6 oz. dark chocolate, chopped
2 tablespoons butter
½ teaspoon vanilla extract
2 teaspoons orange zest
Cocoa powder for serving

Directions:

1. Heat the heavy cream in a saucepan over low heat.
2. Remove from heat and stir in the remaining ingredients.
3. Mix well until smooth and freeze the mixture for 30 minutes or more until well set.
4. Take teaspoons of mixture and form small truffles.
5. Roll them through cocoa powder and serve them.

Meringues

Time: 3 hours
Servings: 2 dozen

Ingredients:

- 4 egg whites
- 1 pinch salt
- 1 teaspoon lemon juice
- 1 cup Splenda
- ½ teaspoon vanilla extract

Directions:

1. Mix the egg whites with salt and lemon juice until fluffy.
2. Gradually add the Splenda and keep mixing until you get a fluffy, stiff meringue.
3. Add the vanilla extract then spoon the meringue into a pastry bag.
4. Pipe small meringues on baking trays lined with parchment paper and cook in the preheated oven at 300F for 2 hours.
5. When done, turn the oven off and let them cool in the oven.

Carrot Cake Loaf

Time: 1 hour
Yields: 1 loaf

Ingredients:

- 1½ cups almond flour
- 1 cup shredded coconut
- 1 teaspoon baking powder
- ½ teaspoon baking soda
- 1 pinch salt
- ½ teaspoon cinnamon powder
- ½ teaspoon ground ginger
- 3 eggs
- ¼ cup Splenda powder
- 1½ cups grated carrot

Directions:

1. Mix the almond flour, coconut, baking powder, baking soda, salt, cinnamon and ginger in a bowl.
2. In a different bowl, combine the eggs with Splenda and mix until frothy.
3. Stir in the flour mixture then fold in the grated carrot.
4. Pour the batter into a loaf pan lined with parchment paper.
5. Bake in the preheated oven at 350F for 30-40 minutes or until a toothpick inserted in the center of the cake comes out clean.
6. Let the loaf cool in the pan before serving.

Mocha Chocolate Mousse

Time: 30 minutes
Servings: 4

Ingredients:

- 4 oz. dark chocolate, chopped
- 3 cups heavy cream
- ¼ cup Splenda
- 2 teaspoons instant coffee
- 1 pinch salt
- 1 teaspoon vanilla extract

Directions:

1. Mix the chocolate with 1 cup heavy cream, Splenda, coffee and a pinch of salt in a bowl and melt them together in the microwave.
2. Mix until smooth then let the mixture come to room temperature.
3. Whip the remaining cream until stiff then fold it into the chocolate mixture.
4. Add the vanilla then pour the mousse into 4 serving glasses and refrigerate until set.
5. Serve the mousse chilled, simple or topped with a dollop of cream or fresh fruits.

Orange Jelly Cheesecake

Time: 2 hours
Servings: 6-8

Ingredients:

Crust:
- 1½ cups almond flour
- 4 tablespoons melted butter

Filling:
- 25 oz. cream cheese
- ½ cup Splenda
- 1 teaspoon vanilla extract
- 1 teaspoon orange zest
- 3 eggs
- ½ cup heavy cream

Orange jelly:
- 1 cup fresh orange juice
- 1 teaspoon agar-agar

Directions:

1. To make the crust, mix the almond flour with butter until well combined.
2. Transfer the mixture in a round cake pan and press it well on the bottom of the pan.
3. For the filling, combine the cream cheese with the rest of the ingredients in a bowl and mix well.
4. Pour the mixture over the curst and bake in the preheated oven at 330F for 40 minutes.
5. When done, remove from the oven and let it cool down.
6. For the jelly, combine the orange juice with agar-agar and bring it to a boil.
7. Remove from heat and let the mixture cool down slightly.

8. Pour the jelly over the cheesecake and refrigerate until set.
9. Serve the cheesecake chilled.

Coffee Granita

Time: 2 hours
Servings: 4-6

Ingredients:

3 cups freshly brewed coffee
½ cup Splenda
1 teaspoon vanilla extract

Directions:

1. Combine all the ingredients in a deep container and mix them well.
2. Place the container in the freezer and freeze it for 4 hours, mixing with a fork every 30 minutes to break the ice crystals.
3. Serve the granita chilled.

Orange Jelly

Time: 3 hours
Servings: 4

Ingredients:

4 cups fresh orange juice
¼ cup Splenda
3 teaspoons gelatin
¼ cup cold water

Directions:

1. Mix the orange juice with Splenda.
2. Bloom the gelatin in the cold water for 10 minutes.
3. Melt the gelatin over a hot water bath for a few seconds then mix it with the orange juice.
4. Pour the mixture into 4 glasses and refrigerate until well set, at least 2 hours.

Quick Banana Ice Cream

Time: 5 hours
Servings: 2-4

Ingredients:

4 ripe bananas, sliced
2 tablespoons cocoa powder
2 tablespoons coconut oil

Directions:

1. Place the banana slices in a freezer bag and freeze at least 4 hours.
2. Transfer the bananas in a blender and add the cocoa powder and coconut oil.
3. Pulse until smooth and creamy.
4. Serve the ice cream right away.

Cheesecake Dessert Cups

Time: 30 minutes
Servings: 4

Ingredients:

4 graham crackers
2 cups cream cheese
¼ cup Splenda powder
1½ cups whipped cream
1 teaspoon vanilla extract
Fresh fruits to serve

Directions:

1. Crush the crackers into fine crumbs and spoon them on the bottom of 4 dessert cups.
2. Mix the cream cheese with Splenda and vanilla then fold in the whipped cream.
3. Spoon the cream cheese over the graham crackers.
4. Top with fresh fruits just before serving.

Cinnamon Muffins

Time: 50 minutes
Servings: 12

Ingredients:

1⅜ cups almond flour
1 teaspoon baking powder
1 pinch salt
⅔ cup Splenda
2 eggs
¼ cup butter, melted
1 teaspoon cinnamon powder
2 green apples, peeled and diced

Directions:

1. Combine the almond flour, baking powder, salt, Splenda, eggs, butter and cinnamon in a food processor and pulse until smooth.
2. Spoon the batter into 12 muffin cups lined with muffin papers.
3. Top each muffin with a few apple dices and bake in the preheated oven at 350F for 20-25 minutes.
4. Let the muffins cool in the pan before serving.

Blueberry Cream Cheese Pancakes

Time: 35 minutes
Servings: 2-4

Ingredients:

2 eggs, beaten
1 cup cream cheese
¼ cup Splenda
½ cup almond flour
¼ cup fresh or frozen blueberries

Directions:

1. Mix the eggs with cream cheese, Splenda and almond flour in a bowl.
2. Fold in the blueberries.
3. Heat a non-stick pan over medium flame.
4. Drop spoonfuls of batter on the hot pan and cook on both sides until well risen and golden brown.
5. Stack them on a platter and serve them warm.

Ricotta Cheesecake

Time: 1¼ hours
Servings: 6-8

Ingredients:

Crust:
1½ cups almond meal
4 tablespoons coconut milk
Filling:
20 oz. ricotta cheese
1 cup heavy cream
2 egg whites
4 eggs
½ cup Splenda powder
1 teaspoon vanilla extract

Directions:

1. Mix the almond meal with coconut milk then transfer the mixture in a round cake pan. Press the crust well into the pan.
2. For the filling, combine all the ingredients in a food processor and mix well.
3. Pour the mixture over the crust and cook in the preheated oven at 330F for 40-45 minutes.
4. Serve the cheesecake chilled.

Pecan Scones

Time: 50 minutes
Servings: 6-8

Ingredients:

1 cup butter, chilled
2 cups ground pecans
1 cup whole wheat flour
½ teaspoon baking powder
1 pinch salt
½ cup dried cranberries
2-4 tablespoons chilled water

Directions:

1. Combine the butter, pecans, flour, baking powder and salt in a food processor and pulse until grainy.
2. Add the cranberries and water just to obtain an easy to work dough.
3. Transfer the dough on your baking tray and shape it into a thick round.
4. Cut the round into triangles and separate them carefully.
5. Cook in the preheated oven at 350F for 20-25 minutes or until golden brown and crisp.
6. Let them cool in the pan before serving.

Mocha Cake

Time: 1 hour
Servings: 6-8

Ingredients:

4 eggs
¼ cup Splenda, granulated
½ teaspoon vanilla extract
¼ cup water
2 cups almond flour
2 tablespoons protein powder
¼ cup cocoa powder
1 teaspoon instant coffee

1 pinch salt

1 teaspoon baking powder

Directions:

1. Mix the eggs with Splenda in a bowl and whip until they double their volume.
2. Add the vanilla and water.
3. Sift the flour with protein powder, cocoa powder, instant coffee, salt and baking powder.
4. Fold the almond flour mixture into the whipped eggs.
5. Pour the batter into a round cake pan lined with parchment paper.
6. Bake in the preheated oven at 350F for 40 minutes.
7. Let the cake cool in the pan before serving.

Coconut Bread

Time: 1 hour
Yields: 1 loaf

Ingredients:

6 eggs
½ cup Splenda
½ teaspoon vanilla extract
1 cup coconut flour
½ cup shredded coconut
1 pinch salt
1 teaspoon baking powder

Directions:

1. Mix the eggs with Splenda until they double their volume.
2. Stir in the vanilla extract then fold in the coconut flour, shredded coconut, salt and baking powder.
3. Pour the batter into a loaf pan lined with parchment paper and bake in the preheated oven at 350F for 30-40 minutes or until well risen and golden brown.
4. Serve the bread warm or chilled.

Lemon Curd

Time: 30 minutes
Servings: 2-4

Ingredients:

½ cup lemon juice
¼ cup Splenda powder
4 egg yolks
2 whole eggs

2 tablespoons lemon zest ¼ cup butter, cubed

Directions:

1. Combine all the ingredients in a heat proof bowl.
2. Place the bowl over a hot water bath and cook for 20 minutes, stirring all the time with a whisk.
3. It is done when it's thick and creamy.
4. When done, remove from the water bath and pass the curd through a fine sieve to remove the zest.
5. Store the curd in a sealed glass jar.

Key Lime Pie

Time: 1½ hours
Servings: 6-8

Ingredients:

Crust:
1 cup pecans
1 cup almonds
3 tablespoons melted butter
Filling:
2 cups heavy cream
3 key lime pies, zested and juiced
4 egg yolks
2 whole eggs
1 pinch salt
1 teaspoon vanilla extract
½ cup Splenda

Directions:

1. For the crust, mix the pecans with almonds in a food processor and pulse until ground.
2. Add the butter and mix well then spoon the mixture on the bottom of a round baking pan and press it well on the bottom and sides of the pan with your fingertips.
3. For the filling, combine all the ingredients in a food processor and pulse until smooth.
4. Pour the mixture into your crust and cook in the preheated oven at 330F for 40-45 minutes or until the center looks set.
5. Let the pie cool in the pan before slicing and serving.

Limoncello Cheesecake

Time: 1¼ hours
Servings: 6-8

Ingredients:

Crust:
1½ cups ground almonds
½ cup ground pecans
3 tablespoons melted butter
Filling:
20 oz. ricotta cheese
5 oz. cream cheese
4 eggs
¼ cup Italian Limoncello
1 teaspoon vanilla extract
1 pinch salt
½ cup Splenda powder

Directions:

1. To make the crust, mix all the ingredients in a food processor and pulse until well mixed.
2. Transfer the mixture in a round cake pan and press it well on the bottom of the pan.
3. To make the filling, mix all the ingredients in a food processor and pulse until smooth.
4. Pour the filling over the crust and cook in the preheated oven at 350F for 40-45 minutes.
5. Let the cheesecake cool in the pan before serving.

Basic Crepes

Time: 40 minutes
Servings: 4-6

Ingredients:

4 eggs, beaten
1½ cups whole milk
1 cup all-purpose flour
4 tablespoons vegetable oil
1 pinch salt

Directions:

1. Combine all the ingredients in a blender and pulse until smooth.
2. Heat a large frying pan over medium flame then pour a few tablespoons of batter in the pan.
3. Toss the pan around to evenly coat the bottom and fry the crepe on both sides until golden brown.
4. Stack the crepes on a platter and serve them filled with your favorite jam, Nutella or fresh fruits.

Berry Cream Cheese Tart

Time: 1 hour
Servings: 6-8

Ingredients:

Crust:
1 cup ground almonds
1 cup ground pecans
¼ cup melted butter
Filling:
2 cups cream cheese
1 cup mascarpone cheese
½ cup Splenda
1 teaspoon vanilla extract
½ cup berry puree
Fresh berries to decorate

Directions:

1. To make the crust, combine the ingredients together then transfer the mixture into a round tart pan and press it well on the bottom and sides of the pan.
2. Cook the crust in the preheated oven at 350F for 15 minutes.
3. Let the crust cool down.
4. For the filling, mix all the ingredients in a bowl until smooth and creamy.
5. Spoon the filling into the crust and refrigerate a few hours.
6. Finish with fresh berries before serving.

Flourless Peanut Butter Cookies

Time: 45 minutes
Servings: 2 dozen

Ingredients:

1 cup smooth peanut butter
1 cup brown sugar
1 teaspoon vanilla extract
1 egg

Directions:

1. Mix the peanut butter with sugar and vanilla until smooth.
2. Add the egg and mix well.
3. Line a baking tray with parchment paper.
4. Drop spoonfuls of batter onto the prepared baking tray.
5. Cook in the preheated oven at 350F for 20 minutes.
6. Let them cool in the pan before serving.

Cream Cheese Raspberry Mousse

Time: 30 minutes
Servings: 4-6

Ingredients:

2 cups cream cheese
½ cup Splenda

2 cups fresh raspberries, pureed
1 cup heavy cream, whipped

Directions:

1. Combine the cream cheese with the Splenda and mix until creamy.
2. Stir in the raspberry puree then fold in the whipped cream.
3. Spoon the mousse into serving glasses and serve it chilled.

Chocolate Dipped Apricots

Time: 25 minutes
Servings: 2-4

Ingredients:

½ cup dark chocolate chips
1 teaspoon coconut oil
6 oz. dried apricots

Directions:

1. Melt the chocolate and coconut oil in a heatproof bowl over a hot water bath.
2. Remove the chocolate from heat then dip each dried apricot into the melted chocolate.
3. Place the apricots on a baking sheet lined with parchment paper and refrigerate until set.
4. Serve them chilled.

Flourless Brownies

Time: 1 hour
Servings: 6-8

Ingredients:

4 oz. dark chocolate, chopped

1 cup butter, softened

1 cup Splenda
4 eggs
½ cup cocoa powder
1 pinch salt

Directions:

1. Mix the chocolate with butter in a heatproof bowl and place over a hot water bath.
2. Melt them together then remove from heat and let the mixture cool down slightly.
3. Stir in the Splenda, followed by eggs, one by one.
4. Fold in the cocoa powder and salt then pour the batter into a small square pan lined with parchment paper.
5. Cook in the preheated oven at 350F for 30 minutes.
6. Let them cool in the pan before slicing and serving.

Blueberry Ice Pops

Time: 4 hours
Servings: 6

Ingredients:

2 cups seedless watermelon
1 lime, juiced
1½ cups fresh blueberries
¼ cup Splenda
1 cup water

Directions:

1. Combine all the ingredients in a blender and pulse until smooth.
2. Pour the mixture into your ice pop molds and freeze at least 3 hours.
3. When done, dip them a few seconds in hot water to make the unmolding easier.
4. Serve them immediately.

Vanilla Orange Popsicles

Time: 4½ hours
Servings: 6

Ingredients:

2 cups fresh orange juice
1 cup plain yogurt
1 cup heavy cream
½ cup Splenda
1 teaspoon vanilla extract
1 tablespoon orange zest

Directions:

1. Combine all the ingredients in a blender and pulse until smooth.
2. Pour the mixture into your ice pop molds and freeze at least 4 hours.
3. Serve them chilled.

Salted Chocolate Pecans

Time: 1 hour
Servings: 10

Ingredients:

3 cups pecan halves
1 cup dark chocolate chips
2 teaspoons sea salt flakes

Directions:

1. Melt the chocolate over a hot water bath or in the microwave.
2. Line a baking tray with parchment paper and place aside.
3. Dip each pecan into the melted chocolate, let it drip off slightly and place it on the prepared baking paper sheet.
4. Sprinkle with a few sea salt flakes and repeat with the remaining pecans.
5. Refrigerate until they are set and serve immediately.

Double Berry Ice Cream

Time: 2 hours
Servings: 4-6

Ingredients:

2 cups half and half
½ cup plain yogurt
¼ cup Splenda

2 cups fresh strawberries, diced
1 cup fresh raspberries

Directions:

1. Mix the half and half with yogurt and Splenda in a bowl.
2. Fold in the fresh berries then pour the mixture into your ice cream maker.
3. Churn according to your machine's instructions and serve the ice cream chilled.

Pretzel Truffles

Time: 2 hours
Servings: 10-12

Ingredients:

1½ cups heavy cream
2 cups dark chocolate chips
½ cup crushed pretzels

Directions:

1. Combine the cream and chocolate in a heatproof bowl and melt them together over a hot water bath or in the microwave.
2. Cover the mixture with a cling film and refrigerate 1 hour until set.
3. Take spoonfuls of mixture and form small balls.
4. Roll each ball through crushed pretzels and serve them right away or store them in the fridge in an airtight container.

Strawberry and Yogurt Cups

Time: 20 minutes
Servings: 4

Ingredients:

½ cup crushed hazelnuts
2½ cups Greek style yogurt
1½ cups fresh strawberries, sliced

Directions:

1. Layer the crushed hazelnuts with yogurt and fresh strawberries in dessert glasses.
2. Serve the cups fresh.

Raspberry Panna Cotta

Time: 3 hours
Servings: 4

Ingredients:

1 tablespoon unflavored gelatin   ¼ cup cold water

2 cups heavy cream
½ cup fresh raspberry puree

☐ cup Splenda

Directions:

1. Bloom the gelatin in cold water for 10 minutes.
2. Mix the cream, raspberry puree and Splenda in a bowl.
3. Melt the gelatin over a hot water bath for a few seconds then stir it into the panna cotta.
4. Pour the panna cotta into 4 dessert cups and refrigerate until set, at least 2 hours.

Quick Microwave Chocolate Cake

Time: 10 minutes
Servings: 1

Ingredients:

¼ cup almond flour
1 tablespoon cocoa powder
¼ teaspoon baking powder
2 tablespoons Splenda

1 pinch salt
¼ teaspoon vanilla extract
1 egg
2 tablespoons melted butter

Directions:

1. Combine all the ingredients in a bowl and mix until smooth.
2. Pour the batter into a mug that can go in the microwave.
3. Cook in the microwave on high power for 1½ minutes, up to 2 minutes.
4. Serve the cake chilled.

Peanut Butter Mousse

Time: 25 minutes
Servings: 4-6

Ingredients:

1½ cups cream cheese, softened
½ cup smooth peanut butter

¼ cup Splenda
1 cup heavy cream, whipped

Directions:

1. Mix the cream cheese with peanut butter and Splenda in a bowl.

2. Fold in the whipped cream then spoon the mousse into individual dessert cups.
3. Refrigerate and serve it chilled.

Pink Grapefruit Sorbet

Time: 2 hours
Servings: 4-6

Ingredients:

3 cups pink grapefruit juice
¼ cup Splenda
½ cup cranberry juice
1 teaspoon vanilla extract

Directions:

1. Mix all the ingredients together.
2. Pour the mixture into your ice cream maker and churn until chilled and set.
3. Serve immediately.

Fudgy Brownies

Time: 1 hour
Servings: 8-10

Ingredients:

½ cup butter, softened
½ oz. dark chocolate, chopped
1 egg
½ teaspoon vanilla extract
1 cup almond flour
½ cup cocoa powder
1 pinch salt
½ teaspoon baking powder

Directions:

1. Mix the butter with chocolate in a heatproof bowl and melt them together over a hot water bath or in the microwave.
2. Remove from heat and let the mixture cool down slightly then stir in the egg and vanilla.
3. Fold in the almond flour, cocoa, salt and baking powder then pour the batter into a small square pan lined with parchment paper.
4. Bake in the preheated oven at 350F for 25-30 minutes.
5. Let them cool completely before slicing into small squares.

Fresh Blueberry Tart

Time: 1 hour
Servings: 6-8

Ingredients:

Crust:
2 cups ground walnuts
2 tablespoons coconut flour
¼ cup melted butter
1 pinch salt
Filling:
1½ cups cream cheese, softened
1 cup sour cream
¼ cup Splenda
1 teaspoon vanilla extract
1 tablespoon lemon zest
1 cup fresh blueberries

Directions:

1. To make the crust, combine all the ingredients in a food processor and pulse until well mixed.
2. Transfer the mixture into a round tart pan and press it well on the bottom and sides of the pan.
3. Bake the crust in the preheated oven at 350F for 15 minutes then let it cool completely.
4. For the filling, mix the cream cheese with sour cream, Splenda, vanilla and lemon then spoon the mixture into your crust.
5. Top with fresh blueberries and serve the tart chilled.

Frozen Bananas Covered in Chocolate

Time: 4 hours
Servings: 4

Ingredients:

2 large bananas
½ cup dark chocolate chips, melted
¼ cup chopped pistachio

Directions:

1. Peel the bananas and cut them in half.
2. Place each half of banana on a wooden skewer and freeze the bananas for at least 2 hours.
3. When frozen, dip each banana half in melted chocolate then roll them through chopped pistachio.

4. Serve immediately.

Watermelon Yogurt Ice Cream

Time: 2 hours
Servings: 4-6

Ingredients:

2 cups seedless watermelon
2 cups Greek style yogurt
2 tablespoons Splenda
1 teaspoon lemon juice

Directions:

1. Combine all the ingredients in a blender and pulse until smooth.
2. Pour the mixture into your ice cream maker and churn according to your machine's instructions.
3. Serve chilled or store in an airtight container in the freezer.

Mini Lemon Cheesecakes

Time: 1 hour
Servings: 12

Ingredients:

Crust:
1½ cups ground pecans
3 tablespoons coconut flour
¼ cup melted butter
1 tablespoon Splenda
Filling:
3 cups cream cheese
1 cup sour cream
3 eggs
½ cup Splenda
1 teaspoon vanilla extract
2 tablespoons lemon zest

Directions:

1. To make the crust, mix all the ingredients in a food processor and pulse until well combined.
2. Spoon the mixture into a muffin pan lined with muffin papers and press it well on the bottom of each muffin cup.
3. For the filling, combine all the ingredients in a bowl and mix well.
4. Spoon the mixture into your muffin cups and cook in the preheated oven at 330F for 25-30 minutes.
5. Serve the cheesecakes chilled.

Microwave Chocolate Lava Cake

Time: 15 minutes
Servings: 1

Ingredients:

1 tablespoon butter
1 tablespoon heavy cream
1 egg
2 tablespoons cocoa powder
2 tablespoons almond flour
1 pinch salt
1 small square dark chocolate

Directions:

1. Mix the butter, cream, egg, cocoa powder, almond flour and salt in a microwave mug.
2. Place the chocolate square into the center of the batter and cook in the microwave on high power for 1½ minutes.
3. Let the cake cool down slightly before serving.

Citrus Pound Cake

Time: 1 hour
Servings: 6-8

Ingredients:

2 cups almond flour
1 cup Splenda
½ teaspoon baking soda
1 teaspoon vanilla extract
1 teaspoon lemon zest
1 teaspoon orange zest
1 cup butter, softened
1 cup sour cream
4 eggs

Directions:

1. Combine all the ingredients in a food processor and pulse until smooth.
2. Keep mixing for 2 minutes then pour the batter into a round cake pan lined with parchment paper.
3. Cook in the preheated oven at 350F for 40 minutes or until golden brown.
4. Let the cake cool in the pan before slicing and serving.

Almond Coconut Cake

Time: 1 hour
Servings: 6-8

Ingredients:

4 eggs
¼ cup Splenda
1¾ cups almond flour
1 cup shredded coconut
1 teaspoon baking powder
¼ cup melted butter

Directions:

1. Mix the eggs with Splenda until fluffy then fold in the almond flour, coconut and baking powder.
2. Drizzle in the melted butter and mix gently.
3. Pour the batter into a round cake pan lined with parchment paper and bake in the preheated oven at 350F for 40 minutes.
4. Let the cake cool completely before slicing and serving.

Peanut Butter Cake

Time: 1 hour
Servings: 6-8

Ingredients:

Cake:
½ cup butter, softened
1 egg
¼ cup smooth peanut butter
1 cup Splenda
1 teaspoon vanilla extract
½ cup sour cream
1¼ cups almond flour
1 teaspoon baking powder
1 pinch salt
Glaze:
3 oz. dark chocolate
2 teaspoons coconut oil

Directions:

1. Combine the butter, egg, peanut butter and Splenda in a bowl and mix until smooth.
2. Stir in the vanilla and sour cream then add the almond flour, baking powder and salt.
3. Spoon the batter into a round cake pan lined with parchment paper and cook in the preheated oven at 350F for 40 minutes.
4. Let the cake cool in the pan then transfer it on a platter.

5. For the glaze, melt the chocolate in a heatproof bowl over a hot water bath then stir in the coconut oil.
6. Drizzle the glaze over the cake and serve it chilled.

Raspberry Almond Crumb Cake

Time: 1¼ hours
Servings: 8-10

Ingredients:

Crust:
2 cups almond flour
☐ cup Splenda
1 pinch salt
¼ cup butter, chilled and cubed
1 egg
Filling:

1½ cups cream cheese
2 cups fresh raspberries
Topping:
1 cup almond flour
¼ cup chilled butter
2 tablespoons Splenda

Directions:

1. To make the crust, mix all the ingredients in a food processor until smooth.
2. Spoon the mixture into a square baking pan lined with parchment paper and spread it well with your fingertips.
3. For the filling, spread the cream cheese over the crust and top with fresh raspberries.
4. For the crumb topping, combine all the ingredients in a bowl and mix until grainy.
5. Spread the topping over the raspberries and cook in the preheated oven at 350F for 40-45 minutes.
6. Cut into small squares when chilled.

Ginger Cookies

Time: 1 hour
Servings: 2 dozen

Ingredients:

½ cup butter, softened
1¼ cups almond flour
⅔ cup Splenda
1 egg
¼ teaspoon baking soda

1 teaspoon ground ginger
¼ teaspoon cinnamon powder

Directions:

1. Combine all the ingredients in a food processor and pulse until well mixed.
2. Form small balls of dough and place them on a baking tray lined with parchment paper.
3. Cook in the preheated oven at 350F for 15-20 minutes.
4. Let them cool in the pan then store them in an airtight container for up to 2 weeks.

Vanilla Butter Cookies

Time: 1 hour
Servings: 2 dozen

Ingredients:

1½ cups almond flour
¼ cup Splenda
¼ cup butter, softened
2 egg whites
1 pinch salt
1 teaspoon vanilla extract

Directions:

1. Combine all the ingredients in a food processor and pulse until well mixed.
2. Freeze the dough for 10 minutes then drop spoonful of dough on a baking tray lined with parchment paper.
3. Cook in the preheated oven at 350F for 15-20 minutes or until the edges begin to turn slightly golden brown.
4. Let the cookies cool in the pan before serving. Store them in an airtight container for up to 2 weeks.

Spiced Cookies

Time: 1 hour
Servings: 2 dozen

Ingredients:

1½ cups almond flour
1 teaspoon ground ginger
2 egg whites
¼ cup Splenda
1 tablespoons dark molasses
1 pinch salt
½ cup granular Splenda
1 teaspoon cinnamon powder

Directions:

1. Combine the almond flour, ginger, egg whites, Splenda, molasses and salt in a food processor.
2. Pulse until well combined then form small balls of dough.
3. Mix the granular Splenda with cinnamon powder in a bowl.
4. Roll each ball through the Splenda and cinnamon mixture and place them on a baking tray lined with parchment paper.
5. Bake in the preheated oven at 350F for 15-20 minutes.
6. Let them cool in the pan then store in an airtight container for up to 2 weeks.

Apple Cheesecake

Time: 1¼ hours
Servings: 6-8

Ingredients:

Crust:
1½ cups ground walnuts
2 tablespoons melted butter
2 tablespoons Splenda
Filling:
3 green apples, peeled and sliced
3 cups cream cheese
1 cup sour cream
3 eggs
⅔ cup Splenda
1 teaspoon cinnamon powder
1 pinch salt
1 teaspoon vanilla extract

Directions:

1. To make the crust, mix the walnuts, butter and Splenda in a bowl.
2. Spoon the mixture into a round cake pan and press it well on the bottom of the pan.
3. Place the apple slices over the crust.
4. Combine the remaining ingredients to make the filling then pour the cheese mixture over the apples.
5. Cook in the preheated oven at 330F for 45 minutes.
6. Let the cheesecake cool in the pan before serving.

Pecan Cookies

Time: 1 hour
Servings: 2 dozen

Ingredients:

3 egg whites
1 pinch salt
⅔ cup Splenda
1 cup almond flour
1 cup ground pecans

Directions:

1. Combine the egg whites with a pinch of salt and whip until fluffy.
2. Add the Splenda and mix until stiff.
3. Fold in the almond flour and pecans then drop spoonfuls of batter on a baking sheet lined with parchment paper.
4. Cook in the preheated oven at 350F for 15-20 minutes or until slightly golden brown.
5. Let the cookies cool in the pan and store them in an airtight container for up to 1 week.

No Bake Cheesecake

Time: 2 hours
Servings: 8-10

Ingredients:

Crust:
1 cup ground almonds
½ cup ground pecans
¼ cup melted butter
Filling:
2 cups cream cheese
½ cup Splenda
1 teaspoon vanilla extract
2 cups heavy cream, whipped
Fresh berries for serving

Directions:

1. To make the crust, mix the almonds, pecans and butter in a bowl.
2. Spoon the mixture into a round cake pan and press it well on the bottom of the pan.
3. For the filling, mix the cream cheese with Splenda and vanilla in a bowl then fold in the whipped cream.
4. Pour the filling over the crust and refrigerate the cheesecake for at least 1 hour.
5. Top the cheesecake with fresh berries before serving.

No Crust Pumpkin Pie

Time: 1 hour
Servings: 6-8

Ingredients:

1 can pumpkin puree
3 eggs
⅔ cup Splenda
1 cup heavy cream
1 teaspoon cinnamon powder
½ teaspoon ground ginger
¼ teaspoon ground cloves
1 pinch salt
1 teaspoon vanilla extract
Butter to grease the pan

Directions:

1. Combine all the ingredients in a blender and pulse until smooth.
2. Grease a round pie pan with butter and pour the pumpkin mixture into the pan.
3. Cook in the preheated oven at 330F for 40-45 minutes.
4. Let the pie cool completely before serving.

No Crust Mocha Cheesecake

Time: 1 hour
Servings: 6-8

Ingredients:

4 cups cream cheese
4 eggs
¼ cup dark cocoa powder
2 teaspoons instant coffee
1 pinch salt
1 teaspoon vanilla extract
¼ cup melted butter
¼ cup almond flour

Directions:

1. Combine all the ingredients in a food processor and pulse until well combined.
2. Pour the batter into a round cake pan lined with parchment paper and cook in the preheated oven at 330F for 45 minutes.
3. Let the cheesecake cool completely before serving.

Chocolate Silk Pie

Time: 1 hour
Servings: 6-8

Ingredients:

Crust:
1½ cups ground walnuts
1 tablespoon coconut flour
1 egg white
2 tablespoons melted butter
Filling:

8 oz. heavy cream
2 tablespoons Splenda
10 oz. dark chocolate, chopped
1 pinch salt
2 tablespoons butter
2 cups heavy cream, whipped

Directions:

1. To make the crust, combine all the ingredients in a food processor and pulse until well mixed.
2. Transfer the mixture in a round pie pan and press it well on the bottom and sides of the pan.
3. Bake the crust in the preheated oven at 350F for 20 minutes.
4. Let the crust cool completely.
5. To make the filling, heat the cream and Splenda in a saucepan.
6. Remove from heat and stir in the chocolate.
7. Mix until melted then add the salt and butter and mix well.
8. Pour the filling over the crust and refrigerate 30 minutes.
9. Top with whipped cream and serve the pie chilled.

Coconut Crisp Cookies

Time: 1 hour
Servings: 2 dozen

Ingredients:

½ cup coconut flour
1 cup shredded coconut
2 egg whites

½ teaspoon vanilla extract
¼ cup Splenda

Directions:

1. Combine all the ingredients in a food processor and pulse until well mixed.
2. Drop spoonfuls of mixture on a baking tray lined with parchment paper and bake in the preheated oven at 350F for 20 minutes or until slightly golden brown.
3. Let the cookies cool in the pan then store them in an airtight container for up to 1 week.

Italian Ricotta Cake

Time: 1 hour
Servings: 6-8

Ingredients:

4 eggs, separated
1 pinch salt
1 cup Splenda
3 cups ricotta cheese
½ cup butter, softened
1 teaspoon lemon zest
1 teaspoon orange zest
1 teaspoon vanilla extract
Butter to grease the pan

Directions:

1. Whip the egg whites with a pinch of salt until stiff. Stir in half of the Splenda and mix until stiff and glossy.
2. Combine the egg yolks, ricotta, butter, lemon zest, orange zest and vanilla in a bowl and mix well.
3. Fold in the whipped egg whites then pour the batter into a round cake pan greased with butter.
4. Bake in the preheated oven at 350F for 40-45 minutes or until slightly golden brown and well risen.
5. Let the cake cool completely before serving.

Hazelnut Coffee Cookies

Time: 1 hour
Servings: 2 dozen

Ingredients:

1 cup ground hazelnuts
2 tablespoons coconut flour
1 teaspoon instant coffee
¼ cup Splenda
2 tablespoons melted butter
1 pinch salt
1 pinch cinnamon powder
1 egg white

Directions:

1. Combine the hazelnuts with coconut flour, coffee, Splenda, butter, salt and cinnamon in a bowl.
2. Whip the egg white until fluffy and fold it into the mixture you just made.
3. Drop spoonfuls of batter on a baking tray lined with parchment paper and bake in the preheated oven at 350F for 20 minutes or until golden brown.

4. Let them cool in the pan before serving.
5. Store in an airtight container for up to 1 week.

Cocoa Flax Cookies

Time: 1 hour
Servings: 2 dozen

Ingredients:

1 cup flax seeds, ground
¼ cup cocoa powder
½ teaspoon baking powder
1 pinch salt

2 eggs
½ teaspoon vanilla extract
2 tablespoons melted butter

Directions:

1. Combine the flax seeds, cocoa powder, baking powder and salt in a bowl.
2. Stir in the eggs, vanilla and butter and mix well.
3. Drop spoonfuls of batter on a baking tray lined with parchment paper and bake in the preheated oven at 350F for 15-20 minutes.
4. Let the cookies cool in the pan before serving. Store them in an airtight container for up to 1 week.

Cottage Cheese Pudding

Time: 1 hour
Servings: 4-6

Ingredients:

4 eggs, beaten
1 cup heavy cream
1½ cup milk

1½ cups cottage cheese
1 teaspoon vanilla extract
½ cup Splenda

Directions:

1. Mix all the ingredients in a bowl.
2. Pour the mixture into a small deep baking pan and bake in the preheated oven at 350F for 25-30 minutes.
3. Let the pudding cool in the pan before serving.

Minty Panna Cotta

Time: 2 hours
Servings: 4

Ingredients:

2 cups heavy cream
½ cup Greek style yogurt
¼ cup Splenda
2 tablespoons mint syrup

¼ teaspoon peppermint extract
1 tablespoon unflavored gelatin
4 tablespoons cold water

Directions:

1. Mix the heavy cream with yogurt, Splenda, mint syrup and peppermint extract.
2. Combine the gelatin and cold water and bloom for 10 minutes.
3. Melt the gelatin and mix it with the cream.
4. Pour the mixture into 4 individual dessert cups and refrigerate at least 1 hour before serving.

Mocha Baked Custard

Time: 1 hour
Servings: 4

Ingredients:

2 cups heavy cream
¼ cup Splenda
2 teaspoons instant coffee

1 pinch salt
5 egg yolks
1 teaspoon vanilla extract

Directions:

1. Combine all the ingredients in a blender and pulse until smooth.
2. Pour the mixture into 4 individual ramekins.
3. Place the ramekins in a deep pan. Pour hot water into the pan, all around the ramekins.
4. Bake in the preheated oven at 330F for 35-40 minutes or until set in the center.
5. Let them cool down before serving.

Coconut Panna Cotta

Time: 2 hours
Servings: 6

Ingredients:

- 1 tablespoon unflavored gelatin
- 4 tablespoons cold water
- 1½ cups coconut milk
- 1½ cups heavy cream
- ½ cup Splenda
- 1 teaspoon coconut extract
- ½ teaspoon vanilla extract

Directions:

1. Bloom the gelatin in cold water for 10 minutes.
2. Mix the coconut milk with cream, Splenda, coconut extract and vanilla in a bowl.
3. Melt the gelatin and mix it into the coconut mixture.
4. Pour the panna cotta in 6 individual serving glasses and refrigerate at least 1 hour until set.

Chocolate Pots de Creme

Time: 1 hour
Servings: 4

Ingredients:

- 1 cup heavy cream
- ¾ cup dark chocolate chips
- 1 pinch salt
- 2½ cups whole milk
- ½ cup Splenda
- 2 egg yolks
- 3 whole eggs

Directions:

1. Mix the cream with chocolate chips in a heatproof bowl and melt them together.
2. Stir in the salt, milk and Splenda, as well as egg yolks and eggs.
3. Pour the mixture into 4 ramekins and cook in the preheated oven at 300F for 40 minutes.
4. Let the pots de creme cool down for 15 minutes before serving.

Beverages

Chocolate Milkshake with Protein Powder

Time: 10 minutes
Servings: 2-4

Ingredients:

2 cups whole milk
1 cup cold water
1 teaspoon peppermint extract
2 tablespoons cocoa powder
2 scoops vanilla protein powder

Directions:

1. Combine all the ingredients in a blender and pulse until smooth.
2. Pour the shake in glasses and serve it chilled.

Chocolate Milkshake

Time: 10 minutes
Servings: 2-4

Ingredients:

½ cup heavy cream
2 cups almond milk
2 tablespoons Splenda
½ teaspoon vanilla extract
4 ice cubes

Directions:

1. Combine all the ingredients in a blender.
2. Pulse until smooth then pour the drink in glasses and serve it fresh.

Strawberry Almond Smoothie

Time: 15 minutes
Servings: 2-4

Ingredients:

1 cup fresh strawberries, halved
2 cups almond milk
2 tablespoons blanched almonds
2 tablespoons Splenda
1 scoop vanilla protein powder

Directions:

1. Combine all the ingredients in a blender.
2. Pulse until smooth then pour the drink in glasses and serve it fresh.

Orange Creamsicle Smoothie

Time: 15 minutes
Servings: 2-4

Ingredients:

2 cups almond milk
1 orange, cut into segments
¼ cup heavy cream
2 scoops vanilla protein powder
½ cup crushed ice

Directions:

1. Combine all the ingredients in a blender and pulse until smooth.
2. Pour the smoothie in glasses and serve it chilled.

Cream Raspberry Sparkler

Time: 10 minutes
Servings: 2-4

Ingredients:

½ cup heavy cream
¼ cup raspberry puree
1½ cups sparkling water

Directions:

1. Combine the ingredients in a jar and shake until mixed.
2. Serve immediately.

Spinach and Parsley Smoothie

Time: 15 minutes
Servings: 2-4

Ingredients:

1 cup low fat yogurt
1 cup almond milk

2 cups fresh spinach
¼ cup fresh parsley
½ teaspoon grated ginger

Directions:

1. Combine all the ingredients in a blender.
2. Pulse until smooth and serve the smoothie fresh.

Grapefruit Spinach Smoothie

Time: 15 minutes
Servings: 2-4

Ingredients:

1 grapefruit, cut into segments
1 cup fresh baby spinach
1 handful fresh parsley
1 cup filtered water
½ cup crushed ice
1 cup low fat yogurt

Directions:

1. Combine all the ingredients in a blender and pulse until smooth.
2. Pour the drink in glasses and serve immediately.

Almond Apple Smoothie

Time: 15 minutes
Servings: 2-4

Ingredients:

1¾ cups almond milk
2 tablespoons blanched almonds
1 green apple, cored and peeled
1 pinch cinnamon powder
½ teaspoon lemon juice

Directions:

1. Combine all the ingredients in a blender and pulse until smooth.
2. Pour the smoothie in glasses and serve it fresh.

Cinnamon Apple Smoothie

Time: 15 minutes
Servings: 2-4

Ingredients:

1½ cups almond milk
2 tablespoons blanched almonds
1 cup crushed ice
1 green apple, peeled and sliced
½ teaspoon lemon juice
½ teaspoon cinnamon powder

Directions:

1. Combine all the ingredients in a blender and pulse until smooth.
2. Pour the smoothie in glasses and serve it fresh.

Avocado Spinach Smoothie

Time: 15 minutes
Servings: 2-4

Ingredients:

½ avocado, frozen
2 cups fresh spinach
1 cup chilled water
1 cup almond milk
¼ cup sunflower seeds
1 lime, juiced

Directions:

1. Combine all the ingredients in a blender and pulse until smooth.
2. Pour the smoothie in glasses and serve it fresh.

Kiwi Smoothie

Time: 15 minutes
Servings: 2-4

Ingredients:

4 ripe kiwi fruits, peeled
4 mint leaves
1 cup fresh spinach
1½ cups almond milk
4 ice cubes

Directions:

1. Mix all the ingredients in a blender.
2. Pulse until smooth then pour the smoothie in glasses and serve it fresh.

Berry Spinach Smoothie

Time: 10 minutes
Servings: 2-4

Ingredients:

1 cup frozen mixed berries
1 cup baby spinach
2 scoops protein powder
1½ cups almond milk
½ cup crushed ice

Directions:

1. Mix all the ingredients in a blender and pulse until smooth.
2. Pour the drink in glasses and serve it as fresh as possible.

Savory Shake

Time: 15 minutes
Servings: 2-4

Ingredients:

1 ripe tomato, peeled and seeded
¼ cup fresh parsley
¼ cup fresh cilantro
1 small cucumber, peeled
1 jalapeño pepper, seeded
1 cup filtered water
½ cup crushed ice

Directions:

1. Mix all the ingredients in a blender.
2. Pulse until smooth then pour the shake into glasses and serve it as fresh as possible.

Coconut Vanilla Shake

Time: 10 minutes

Servings: 2-4

Ingredients:

2 cups low fat coconut milk
4 tablespoons vanilla protein powder

½ teaspoon vanilla extract

4 ice cubes

Directions:

1. Mix all the ingredients in a blender and pulse until smooth.
2. Pour the shake in glasses and serve it chilled.

Green Smoothie

Time: 15 minutes
Servings: 2-4

Ingredients:

2 cups fresh spinach
1 cup crushed ice
1 cup almond milk

½ ripe avocado
1 scoop vanilla protein powder

Directions:

1. Combine all the ingredients in a blender and pulse until smooth.
2. Pour the smoothie in glasses and serve it as fresh as possible.

Berry Yogurt Shake

Time: 10 minutes
Servings: 2-4

Ingredients:

¾ cup mixed berries
1½ cups plain yogurt

1 cup filtered water
4 ice cubes

Directions:

1. Combine all the ingredients in a blender.
2. Pulse until smooth then pour in glasses and serve it chilled.

Banana Mocha Shake

Time: 10 minutes
Servings: 2-4

Ingredients:

1 small ripe banana
1½ cups almond milk
1 cup filtered water
2 tablespoons cocoa powder
1 teaspoon instant coffee
½ teaspoon vanilla extract

Directions:

1. Combine all the ingredients in a blender and pulse until smooth.
2. Pour the shake in glasses and serve it as fresh as possible as it tends to change color and lose nutrients.

Chilled Mango Smoothie

Time: 10 minutes
Servings: 2-4

Ingredients:

6 ice cubes
1½ cups plain yogurt
½ mango, sliced
½ cup filtered water
1 scoop vanilla protein powder

Directions:

1. Combine all the ingredients in a blender.
2. Pulse until smooth then pour the drink in glasses and serve it chilled.

Kiwi Yogurt Shake

Time: 15 minutes
Servings: 2-4

Ingredients:

4 kiwi fruits, peeled
1 cup plain yogurt
½ cup filtered water
½ cup crushed ice
1 tablespoon flax seeds

Directions:

1. Combine all the ingredients in a blender.
2. Pulse until smooth then pour the drink in glasses and serve it fresh.

Vanilla Hot Chocolate

Time: 20 minutes
Servings: 4-6

Ingredients:

½ cup dark chocolate chips
1 cup heavy cream
1½ cups hot water
2 tablespoons cocoa powder
1 teaspoon vanilla extract
2 tablespoons Splenda

Directions:

1. Combine the chocolate chips and cream in a saucepan and melt them together over low heat.
2. Stir in the remaining ingredients and mix well.
3. Pour the drink in glasses and serve it fresh.

Mexican Hot Chocolate

Time: 15 minutes
Servings: 2-4

Ingredients:

1½ cups almond milk
1 cup heavy cream
2 tablespoons cocoa powder
2 tablespoons Splenda
¼ teaspoon cinnamon powder
¼ teaspoon cayenne pepper

Directions:

1. Combine all the ingredients in a saucepan.
2. Place over low heat and bring to the boiling point, mixing until smooth.
3. Pour in glasses and serve immediately.

Sugar Free Hot Chocolate

Time: 15 minutes
Servings: 4-6

Ingredients:

3 tablespoons cocoa powder
½ cup hot water
2 cups whole milk
1 pinch cinnamon powder

Directions:

1. Combine all the ingredients in a saucepan.
2. Bring to the boiling point over low heat and mix until smooth.
3. Pour the drink in glasses and serve it warm.

Spiced Hot Cocoa

Time: 20 minutes
Servings: 4-6

Ingredients:

¼ cup dark cocoa powder
2 tablespoons Splenda
¼ teaspoon cinnamon powder
1 pinch salt
¼ teaspoon ground cloves
1 pinch cayenne pepper
3 cups milk
½ teaspoon vanilla extract

Directions:

1. Combine all the ingredients in a saucepan.
2. Bring the mixture to the boiling point, mixing well with a whisk until smooth.
3. Pour the drink in glasses and serve it hot.

Peanut Butter Smoothie

Time: 10 minutes
Servings: 2-4

Ingredients:

1½ cups low fat milk
½ ripe banana
2 tablespoons smooth peanut butter
1 pinch cinnamon

Directions:

1. Combine all the ingredients in a blender and pulse until smooth.
2. Pour the smoothie in glasses and serve it fresh.

Grapefruit Kale Juice

Time: 10 minutes
Servings: 2-4

Ingredients:

3 pink grapefruits
6 kale leaves

Directions:

1. Juice all the ingredients and mix the juice well.
2. Serve the juice as fresh as possible.

Cantaloupe Yogurt Smoothie

Time: 10 minutes
Servings: 2-4

Ingredients:

2 cups cantaloupe cubes
1 cup plain yogurt
1 cup crushed ice
1 tablespoon Splenda

Directions:

1. Combine all the ingredients in a blender.
2. Pulse until smooth then pour the smoothie in glasses and serve it fresh.

Pineapple Milkshake

Time: 15 minutes
Servings: 2-4

Ingredients:

1 cup fresh pineapple cubes
1 cup plain yogurt
1 cup almond milk
2 scoops vanilla protein powder

Directions:

1. Combine all the ingredients in a blender and pulse until smooth and creamy.
2. Pour the milkshake in glasses and serve it as fresh as possible.

Nectarine Smoothie

Time: 15 minutes
Servings: 2-4

Ingredients:

3 ripe nectarines, pitted and sliced
½ cup Greek style yogurt
1½ cups almond milk
½ cup crushed ice
1 tablespoon Splenda
½ teaspoon orange zest

Directions:

1. Combine all the ingredients in a blender.
2. Pulse until smooth and then pour the drink in glasses and serve it as fresh as possible.

Tropical Smoothie

Time: 15 minutes
Servings: 2-4

Ingredients:

1 cup fresh pineapple cubes
1 teaspoon grated ginger
½ papaya
1½ cups almond milk
½ cup crushed ice

Directions:

1. Combine all the ingredients in a blender and pulse until smooth.
2. Pour the smoothie in glasses and serve it as fresh as possible as it tends to lose nutrients in time.

Plum Tangerine Juice

Time: 10 minutes
Servings: 2-4

Ingredients:

6 ripe plums, pitted
4 tangerines

Directions:

1. Juice all the ingredients then mix the juices together.
2. Serve the juice as fresh as possible as it tends to lose nutrients in time.

Low Carb Lemonade

Time: 15 minutes
Servings: 4-6

Ingredients:

5 cups filtered water
6 ice cubes
2 lemons, sliced
1 lemon, juiced
½ cup Splenda

Directions:

1. Combine all the ingredients in a glass jar.
2. Serve the lemonade fresh and chilled.

Pink Lemonade

Time: 15 minutes
Servings: 4-6

Ingredients:

1 lemon, peeled and cut into segments
1 lemon, juiced
1 cup fresh strawberries
5 cups filtered water
1 cup crushed ice
½ cup Splenda

Directions:

1. Mix the strawberries and lemon in a blender and pulse until smooth.
2. Stir in the remaining ingredients and serve the lemonade fresh.

Raspberry Yogurt Smoothie

Time: 10 minutes
Servings: 2-4

Ingredients:

1 cup fresh raspberries
1 cup plain yogurt
1½ cups almond milk
½ teaspoon vanilla extract
1 tablespoon blanched almonds

Directions:

1. Combine all the ingredients in a blender.
2. Pulse until smooth then pour the smoothie in glasses and serve it as fresh as possible.

Conclusion

The world we live in may not be the healthiest, but you still have a choice for a healthy lifestyle and diet. And the more you delay making this change, the more your body and mind lose! So wait no more and go low carb now! It's time to overcome your body's addictions to sugars and starches and restart your system completely. It's time to lose those stubborn pounds and improve your lifestyle. It may not be easy, but it sure is rewarding!

Thank you again for purchasing this book!

Finally, if you enjoyed this book, please take the time to share your thoughts and post a review on Amazon. It'd be greatly appreciated!

Feel free to contact me at emma.katie@outlook.com

Check out more books by Emma Katie at:

www.amazon.com/author/emmakatie

Made in the USA
Monee, IL
16 August 2023

41127556R00109